Edited by Donald Holden
Designed by William Harris
Composed in Twelve Point Century Expanded

HOW TO
LOSE
WEIGHT
WELL

Keep weight off forever, the healthy, simple way

DR XAND VAN TULLEKEN

Photography by Louise Hagger and Colin Bell

quadrille

Health warnings

Seriously considering your weight and your reasons for losing weight can play havoc with your self-confidence. When you're struggling, give yourself a hug, have a cup of tea and a cry. That's what I do. It's hard work and you deserve love and praise for trying. There are other specific health issues around weight loss. If you're concerned about the effect of dieting on your health, seek help from your general practitioner or the practice nurse. I know this isn't always convenient so it's always worth considering seeing a dietitian. You can see them on the NHS or privately, depending on your needs and means. Dietitians are trained and licensed; nutritionists aren't. Anyone can call themselves a nutritionist.

▶ You shouldn't be trying to lose weight if you are underweight or you have, or suspect you have, an eating disorder (including anorexia and bulimia). If you have any history of psychiatric illness I think you should seek advice from your GP or at least from a dietitian so that you have someone to check up on you.

▶ If you are under 18 years of age, even if you are overweight, you should seek advice from your GP or from a qualified dietitian. The long-term health consequences of dieting badly when you're young are hard to overstate.

▶ If you are pregnant or breastfeeding, you should discuss any plans to lose weight with your doctor.

▶ If you are frail in any way (recovering from major illness or surgery), again, I'd strongly advise that you consult your GP or a dietitian.

▶ If you are on any medication, check with your GP or pharmacist.

▶ If you are an insulin-dependent or Type-1 diabetic, review any weight-loss plans with your care team.

▶ If you are actively unwell (fever or other symptoms of illness), this is not the right time to start dieting.

▶ Finally, salt. If you cook at home and you're losing weight then it's unlikely you'll be having too much salt. Even if you have quite a bit the weight loss should offset its effects. But some people respond worse to salt than others. If you're a heavy salt user or you're concerned about your health, get your blood pressure checked.

DO NOT ASK IF I AM BEACH BODY READY

O do not ask
if I am beach body ready.

Observe how the folds
of my stomach ripple
like the wind-pulled waves.

Feel these pale buttocks,
smoothed by the sand-grains
of time.

Note these milk-white limbs,
useless and stranded,
washed up whalebones.

Consider the tufts of hair
which sprout on my shoulders
like sea-grass.

And listen to the lapping
of my socks
at the shores of my sandals.

And you ask me
if I am beach body ready?

BRIAN BILSTON

CONTENTS

INTRODUCTION

WHAT DOES IT MEAN TO 'LOSE WEIGHT WELL'?

I think for most people it's something like: "I want to lose my excess fat quickly, easily and healthily. Oh, and actually I don't mind it being unhealthy... and it doesn't need to be that easy – provided it really works I'll try anything. Oh, and also, I don't really care about weight – I just want to be able to fit into smaller clothes and look good naked. Please just make me thinner, you know, like a supermodel or a movie star." Different people want slightly different things but I'm guessing if you're reading this it means you'd like to look 'thinner'.

I can definitely help you do this, and let's be ambitious about this goal: I don't want you just to be thinner. I want you to be healthy in every sense of the word; I want you to lose weight in the form of fat not muscle; and I'd like it to be as easy as possible.

So, we have a simple goal:
lose weight, be healthy, and find a
way of doing this that is possible for
a normal human being.

I think most people would say that achieving this goal would be worth the price of admission. But let me go further: this book is aimed at helping you achieve a really difficult ambition. Losing weight is hard. Hard like world peace or nuclear physics. Don't take my word for it. The people at Stanford University in the US are pretty smart. The most popular class at that university is called Designing Your Life. It's taught by two rock-star professors and it's so amazing at helping students find their way in the world that other professors also sign up to take it. There are only two issues they say the class can't help you with: finding love and, you guessed it, losing weight. Losing weight is about fighting an extremely basic human urge: the desire to eat. The tools that you need to lose weight will help you tackle other issues in your life as well. It will be impossible to lose weight without taking control of your life. I want to help you do that.

The dream is to lose the weight you want quickly and then maintain it. The book describes four steps to achieve this. Life does get in the way of this dream though: you change jobs, children come along, you get married, divorced, move house, get depression and many other things. All of these things affect our ability to resist temptation or to adopt and stick to regular

> There's no single diet out there that works for everyone. Everyone is different, and everyone's life changes constantly. This book helps you tailor-make a diet that works for you and your life.

habits. I find myself eating ice cream and doughnuts for one reason or another and I have to lose weight that I previously managed to lose and then regained. It's predictable but it's also annoying. So I want to help you lose weight and keep it off and because we're human the plan I've made allows for setbacks.

BODY SHAMING & SEXISM

There's something vaguely uncomfortable for me about writing a diet book. Though I don't say it explicitly anywhere, there's a strong implication that I think you should slim down and tone up. So I'll be as clear as I can. I don't believe you'll look better thinner. I think you might feel better, your feet and knees will hurt less and you'll live longer. And as you lose weight you'll find other parts of your life become easier because of the skills you've learned to get there. You may even, for a host of reasons, find yourself easier to love. That makes it easier to love people around you and have happy relationships with them. But they won't love you any more than they already do because you're thin. And neither will I. I also won't judge you for prioritizing

the cake over the waistline; after all, you could get hit by a bus tomorrow. But if you do eat the cake, do it consciously and after some thought about your life and motivations.

So please don't let any part of this book make you feel bad about yourself. Up close, everyone – supermodel or not – is covered in pores and in-growing hairs and broken veins, with flatulence and morning breath. Don't aim for magazine-fresh perfection. It doesn't exist. The only creatures that are as good in real life as they look on the internet are cats.

POVERTY

Poverty and obesity are closely linked. The poorest areas of the UK have the highest rates of obesity. I wish this book could be aimed at those families and in writing about 'changing your life' I am conscious that for many people this is an impossibility. Unemployment, lack of opportunity and low social mobility mean that the kind of changes that make losing weight an achievable goal are very difficult for many people. I don't think this book is a solution to the obesity crisis, which is to a great extent a product of factors beyond many people's control. I think anyone can lose weight well and take more control of their life but that will be harder for some people than for others. You have my love and support.

This book is arranged around
FOUR BASIC STEPS

1 IDENTIFY AND ELIMINATE YOUR ENEMIES: there are people, organizations and things that want to make you fat or keep you fat. Prepare to do battle. (See page 23.)

2 PREPARE TO EAT WELL: it's hard to know where to start on your own. So I've made you a list. (See page 34.)

3 EAT WELL: hunger is a big problem if you're trying to lose weight. Your body will put up a fight. There are foods that will help you fight back. These are foods that won't induce cravings and will keep you healthy in many other ways. I've written it all down for you. (See page 37.)

4 LIVE WELL: if you're trying to lose weight you'll meet a lot of people who say "all you need to do is diet and exercise". This is annoying and unhelpful. No one struggles to lose weight because they're lazy or stupid. The three steps above are hard and most of us have good reasons for not doing them. In this section I have some advice about how to examine and adjust your entire life to help you lose weight well. (See page 44.)

I'M NO EXPERT...

Well, I am actually kind of an expert. I have a bunch of letters after my name. But my most important qualification for writing this book (I think) is that I have lost a substantial amount of weight and kept it off for a long period of time. I ate my way from 12½ stone to 19 stone over the course of a very stressful 2009. I have weighed less than 13 stone since 2012. Of course, evangelizing about my own weight loss is boring and annoying, and what worked for me won't work for everyone, but this book is written from personal experience.

But about those letters after my name... I studied medicine at Oxford University and I have a degree in public health from Harvard University. When I started trying to lose weight I was lucky that I had enough medical knowledge to approach the problem sensibly. I've tried to put the stuff I found helpful into this book.

> As well as my personal experience with weight loss, I've looked into just about every diet out there.

And I mean I've really looked, not for myself but out of professional interest. I didn't just skim the magazines in the supermarket checkout queue and browse the 'diet books' section at the book shop. I went the extra mile. In fact I went several extra miles: I went right down the rabbit hole and into the crazy world of the diet industry. I bought and read just about every diet book on the market; I looked into every fad; I tried a bunch of the really weird stuff; and I helped contributors on the *How to Lose Weight Well* show with most of the major diet plans out there. I don't know any other doctors who have done this: the world of fad dieting gets little serious scrutiny from the medical profession. I think I can reasonably say that I've reviewed the claims of just about any diet book you could find on the high street.

The rest of my career has involved various aspects of 'extreme nutrition' as well. I can discuss the ideas in the 'paleo diet' books because I've lived with hunter-gatherer tribes in South America, Africa and the Arctic. I can talk about low-carb diets because I've not only read the medical research, I've interviewed the world experts and I've done extreme low-carb dieting myself.

This book draws on over a decade of research, interviews, documentary making and painstaking examination of the scientific literature and dieting advice out there. It also draws on my personal experience of dieting, weight loss, weight gain, cooking and eating.

You've got food companies, the diet industry, the messy science, the media, the internet and of course your own basic human desire to stuff your face with delicious food, all working against you. This book is my attempt to undo this, to simplify things and to help you lose weight without danger to your health, bank balance or overall wellbeing. I hope that it will make your life easier.

Perhaps most importantly, I understand how much life gets in the way of losing weight well. I'm a parent and I'm greedy; I've been unemployed, worked night shifts, travelled a lot and held a desk job. I'm as easily seduced by a fad diet as anyone else and I'm as prone to getting fat as anyone else. I don't believe this is easy, and I don't believe it's your fault that you're in a position where you want to lose weight. I do believe, however, that anyone can get to the weight they want without endangering their health or suffering too much.

I wanted to write a book with diet rules that would work for everyone all of the time. This book is the best of everything I've learned: a collection of ideas that I've begged, borrowed or adapted… or learned the hard way.

WHY IS IT SO EASY TO GAIN WEIGHT?

NEW FOODS

The first problem you face is new foods. By this I mean foods that didn't exist a few decades ago; foods that have been specially designed to make you eat much more of them than you need or even want to. The existence of these foods should be no surprise. After all, if you were a food manufacturer, wouldn't you hire scientists to invent food that was irresistibly delicious? The tastier the food you manufacture, the more people eat. And the more they eat, the more they buy, which is the whole point of running a food company. Well, the big food companies did hire scientists and the results are a range of foods that are 'hyperdelicious' and almost impossible to stop eating: chocolate bars, crisps, ice creams, frozen meals and much, much more.

A couple of years ago I did an experiment with a friend of mine who is an obesity researcher in Philadelphia. She wired up my eyeball so that we could measure the effects of different kinds of food on my brain's reward system. Broccoli and even dark chocolate were fine: my brain enjoyed them but nothing more. Milk chocolate though? That stuff hit my brain like cocaine: we saw a huge spike of dopamine – the brain's reward

In all of human history there has never been a worse time to try to lose weight.

chemical – that lasted about 90 seconds; an intense surge of pleasure followed by longing as the dopamine level returned to normal. Have you ever had the experience of putting the ice cream back in the freezer after what you've absolutely promised yourself is the final, final mouthful, and then almost without thinking about it finding yourself back at the freezer, spoon in hand, a minute and a half later? That isn't your lack of willpower – that's your dopamine levels going crazy. And the food scientists made that happen.

In the case of milk chocolate and ice cream there seemed to be a common mechanism: the ratio of fat to sugar was about 50:50. But food design gets far more complex than that to give you that 'just can't stop' feeling. The ratio of fat, sugar, salt and other chemical flavourings delivered with the right amount of crunch, creaminess, chunkiness, and chewiness means that modern foods are working on your caveman/woman brain and it can't cope. These new foods are making us fatter because we can't resist them.

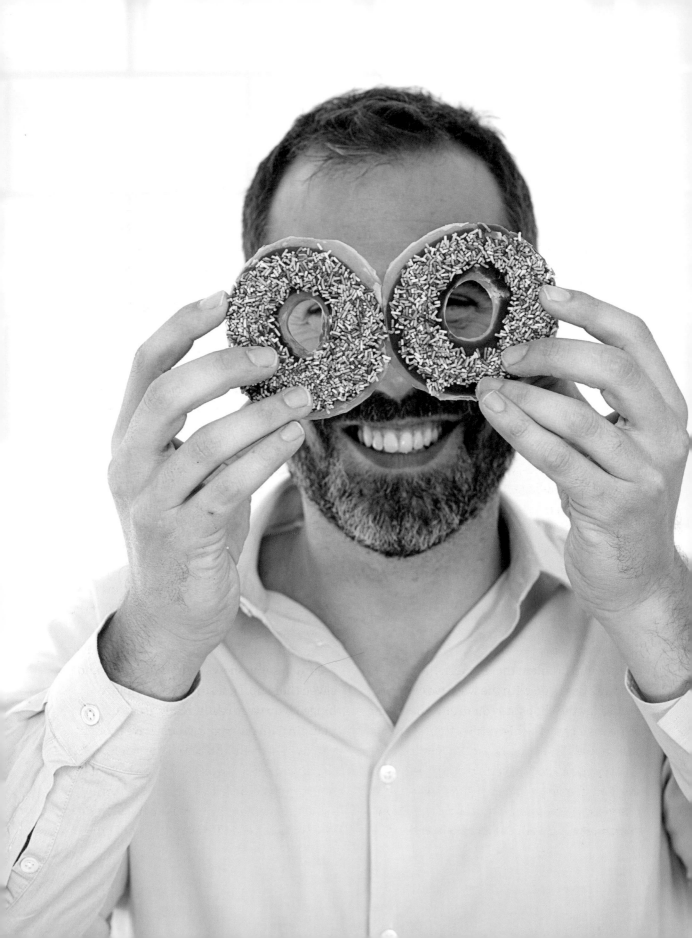

Five hundred years ago two medieval peasants with different abilities to resist tasty food would have been the same weight. Because there wasn't much food around and what there was wasn't very tasty unless you love turnips. But the modern world is not designed for those of us who consider eating a source of real pleasure. We are confronted with abundant, scientifically engineered temptation. This is the main reason that 'junk food' is bad for you: it's not just easy to eat a lot of it, it makes you eat too much of it.

The bottom line is, you can't take any health or weight-loss advice from a large (or even a small) corporation that manufactures food. They don't want you to lose weight. They don't want you to be healthy. They just want you to spend money. And they're very good at what they do.

THE INTERNET

The second problem that modern life presents has to do with the ways we can now eat. Today the shops stay open late, there's far more variety on the high street than ever before, and there is apparently a new by-law that says that every public space in the UK must contain at least two different kinds of pasty shop (and every terminal train station must contain three). But there is one giant change that has opened up entirely new opportunities for weight gain. The internet. Why? Because the internet gloriously allows us to binge on two things at once: food and television (and frequently food-television). The combination of these two delights has been around for decades but now it's different. You can have as much of both as you want, exactly when you want it and it's all amazing. Twenty years ago neither the food nor the television was abundant enough or good enough or varied enough to build a weekend around. Now it is hard to think of any activity that can seriously compete with twelve hours of Scandinavian crime drama (or your favourite American sitcom, wildlife documentary or whatever your particular weakness is) combined with whatever kind of Chinese, Thai, Indian or other culinary wonders your local takeaway will send at the click of a mouse.

Oh, certainly in the old days you could have recorded some shows over a few weeks and saved them up. I guess it was possible to binge if you were really, really great at planning. But everyone would have thought you were extremely odd and the stack of VHS tapes would have been hard to hide. Now it's not just much easier, it's also much more socially acceptable. There is an entire style of online dating called 'Netflix and chill'. You meet a date online and agree to hang out and watch TV and snack. There are commentators who will insist that this is a euphemism for other kinds of date activity. I don't believe them. I think it's the ultimate pitch for a low-pressure, enjoyable evening. Ask my girlfriend.

So the food is too tasty and too abundant and the ways to enjoy it are too numerous. That would seem to account for many of our problems. But all of this could be overcome with sheer willpower, surely. Have we all just become softer and more feeble?

A WORD ON WILLPOWER

The popular perception of people who are overweight is that they lack willpower. This is nonsense.

'Willpower' is a hard concept to understand. When I was at 19 stone, did I have less willpower than I do now (at 13 stone)? And if so, where did the new willpower come from? Does a hard-working business owner who stays up all night working on running the company, resisting every temptation to quit or take a shortcut, have no willpower just because they're overweight? What about the lazy stoners whose sole achievement is staying thin? Are they models of iron will? (No. And no offence to fat businessmen or lazy stoners.)

> There are many people who demonstrate vast amounts of willpower in many parts of their life who can't lose weight.

In the end, willpower is a combination of two things. The first is impulse control. You know that almost automatic feeling of reaching for a brownie or a packet of crisps as if it's a magnet and your hand is made of steel? If you do resist, that's impulse control. Impulse control affects many areas of our lives: it's about resisting temptation in loads of different ways. Sex, drugs, booze, video games, checking social media and so on. The bad news is, it's a little bit genetic. The good news? You can train it. There are apps which will help train your brain to not move your hand towards the cake. And if you sit and stare at the chocolates on the desk and don't reach for them one day, the next day it'll get a little easier.

The second ingredient in willpower is motivation and it's far more important than whatever genetic ability you were born with to resist temptation. Anyone can resist the cake or ice cream if they're told that they'll be paid £1,000. Except the billionaire. That person might just say: "Screw it, I'll have the cake. I don't care about the money." Weddings are a great incentive to lose weight because you know you'll be on display, you've already ordered your outfit and that photo will be on the mantelpiece forever. But it's a motivation that evaporates on the first day of the honeymoon. It's a great kickstart but the best motivation, if you can find it in yourself, is a desire to change in a more fundamental way.

TOTAL CONFUSION AND PARANOIA

Third problem: even if you wanted to restrain yourself and really try to eat healthily, and you have a will of iron, it's still very hard to know what you should eat. This isn't just bad luck. There are many people making things eliberately difficult for you.

If you've ever spent any time asking "how can I lose weight?" you'll know that the thousands of books, websites, DVDs, magazines, corporations, scientists, gurus and others provide endless answers that create a confusing, contradictory mess. Is breakfast important? Should I wash everything down with apple cider vinegar? Do calories matter or should I concentrate on cutting carbs? What about gluten? Did I waste my money on this blender? Look into any of these questions and you'll find not just a total lack of consensus but wild, angry arguments. This is strange because the things involved are not really very complicated. Compared to questions like "how should I raise my children, or make more money," you'd think that agreeing on what to eat and how to exercise in order to feel good, look good and live long wouldn't be too hard. And yet here I am writing a book about it because I think the other sources of information are pretty hopeless.

WHO IS MAKING IT CONFUSING?

▶ **Let's start with scientists.** They should have your back, right? Wrong! (This isn't just some doctor/scientist rivalry talking – although doctors are scientifically more trustworthy.) If you followed the scientific advice on how to eat healthily over the last few decades, you've been seriously misled. Advice to eat margarine, avoid animal fat, reduce egg consumption and consume a low-fat diet has all now been challenged and I think largely overturned. The advice for weight loss and healthy eating has been not just unclear but actively wrong.

Why do scientists get it wrong so often? I think there are three main reasons. The first is that there are huge amounts of money at stake for various industries. If you look at the scientific research investigating the potential harms and benefits of eating fat and sugar, you find that much of it was funded

> I think I can fit everything you need to know about how to eat well and lose weight into this pretty short book and I'm not getting money from any food advertisers.

either by the sugar industry or by the dairy industry. And unsurprisingly each side of this debate advocates either a low-fat diet or a low-sugar diet. All nutrition research is expensive to do because the health effects we're looking for are subtle, take years to reveal themselves, and require huge numbers of people to take part in the trial. So there just isn't much research out there that wasn't paid for by someone with a very particular interest in the answer.

▶ **The second reason I think the advice has been very confusing around what to eat is that we imagine specific foods to have specific effects on our bodies.**
For example, fat makes you fat. Seems reasonable? It's an intuitive proposition and an appealing one. Just like a low-fat diet must surely make low-fat people. Also, not true. A bag of boiled sweets has no fat at all but I strongly recommend you don't think of it as weight-loss food.

▶ **The third reason is that scientists have been limited by the need for simplicity.**
Governments and health professionals want to be able to provide simple advice for their populations that is easy to follow: 5-a-day, low-fat, and so on. The majority of people prefer to eat junk food that is cheap and accessible. So governments oversimplify and set the bar low. This means anyone seriously interested in how to eat and seeking help from, for example, the NHS website, gets advice that is vague, designed not to seriously offend any large corporations, and unambitious. Even when the scientists have been right, the only way for most people to encounter the results of their research is through the media. The media want scoops, splashes and sensational stuff. In order to sell the most papers and magazines, they tell us what we want to hear: quick fixes exist, new fads work, there are miracle weight-loss foods and so on.

I have only encountered one reliable source of good eating advice, despite many years of reading all kinds of literature on the subject – an American journalist named Michael Pollan. His work isn't specifically aimed at weight loss but at a combination of health, environmental and social concerns. He wrote a book called *Food Rules* and I agree with every one of them. His work displays reasonable, thought-through common sense.

BEFORE WE BEGIN

The most important stage of losing weight and keeping it off is a commitment to change. I don't mean changing your weight, I mean changing the things in your life that have made you gain weight. Many of the changes are external, by which I mean they're practical, physical things you can alter about your life. You might need to take the ice cream out of the freezer, or change the timing of your meals for example. I can help with all those decisions and plans. But there is one change you need to commit to that's internal: you need to change how you think of yourself and believe that you can do this. I can't do that for you, and neither can anyone else. You need to find the switch that turns on your motivation to lose weight and your belief that you can do it. I'll try to help you get there with a few questions.

WHY AM I TRYING TO LOSE WEIGHT *NOW*?

In *How to Lose Weight Well* I always ask contributors this question. It's really important to identify what your reasons are because your motivation has a huge effect on your chances of success.

The most common reason people give for wanting to lose weight is an event, such as a wedding, a school reunion or an upcoming beach holiday. All of these are great motivators while they last, but there's a downside to that as motivation: they might kickstart your diet but they will eventually pass, and you can (at least in the case of a party) either stop caring or cancel. Is it a good enough incentive? One event on one day, one group of people whose opinion you may or may not decide to care about? For some people, this may not be enough.

What about just looking better in general? Maybe this is a good enough reason to lose weight? Most people do want to look better after all, and the rewards seem potentially vast. Perhaps you want to stay attractive to your partner or you want to find love. This seems like a great motivation, and I've certainly felt conscious of my weight when I'm dating or with someone I care about. But in reality the people we love usually won't love us more if we shed a few pounds. We can prioritize (or de-prioritize) the importance of looking better for other people on any given day.

Other reasons that I typically hear from people wanting to lose weight are to do with health: "I want to be around longer for my family." This is a great reason but maybe not a great motivator. Most people have trouble imagining themselves sick, or worse, dead, and it's difficult to think about events in the distant future. In the end it's not too hard to put off change for another day.

Other motivations to lose weight include wardrobe issues, snoring, backache or indigestion, and many others. Perhaps your knees ache or your sex life has got worse. It may be a combination of all of these (in which case I'm sorry!). But all of these motivations are susceptible to being abandoned. You can bail on any of them pretty easily – you can buy new trousers, not go to the school reunion and decide that your family isn't worth the effort it would take to stay alive for another few years.

Use any or all of the above motivations if you like. They all kind of worked for me: I hated how I looked, I had a mountain of clothing I could no longer wear, and my blood pressure and my blood sugar were soaring.

But there's an even better motivation: a desire to be a different person, to really change who you are, and to represent this change to the outside world by taking control of your weight. This might sound a little grandiose: "I'm only trying to fit into a cocktail dress for my cousin's wedding!" Well, maybe.

> But you can always buy another dress. You can't buy another you and you should be the best version of yourself you can be.

WHY AM I OVERWEIGHT?

Sometimes it's as simple as asking yourself "where are my excess calories coming from?" and for some people, answering this is pretty easy. If you go to the pub every night and have six pints and a few packets of pork scratchings, the answer is obvious.

But if you have a salad every day for lunch, it's harder.

I recommend that everyone keep a food diary. Without this it's very hard to identify the main problems. You want to keep track of everything you're putting in your mouth: fizzy drinks, snacks, office baked goods, sugar in tea and coffee. Link each entry to a time of day.

Your food diary will help you identify your particular weakness (chocolate, ice cream, etc.) and make a plan to reduce it or work around it. Many people don't have any idea what their weakness is until they look into it – because it's stuff they have so often that it's completely normal. Other people think they have lots of weaknesses because there's lots they enjoy. But I'm talking here about your personal crack; whatever it is that you cannot stop your hand reaching out for.

WHAT ARE THE MAIN BARRIERS TO MY SUCCESS?

There is a fundamental rule of changing your life: all change will be resisted. There's a reason that you are the way you are, and that your world is the way it is. It's either easy or convenient, or it reflects the wishes of most of the people around you.

And they won't like it when you reject their gifts or stop going to the pub with them. They will also probably resent you getting thinner and making them look comparatively fatter. And they won't take any of this lying down.

More importantly, the big food companies won't appreciate you stopping buying their products, so they will market stuff more aggressively than ever. OK, they won't be

Losing weight, however much you'd like it to be a private affair, isn't. People expect you to eat and socialize; people bring food as gifts; people expect you to drink at events you'd normally drink at.

annoyed at you personally, but it will feel that way. Once you're losing weight, you'll really notice the number of free chocolate bars with magazines, the two-for-one pasty deals and the endless TV ads.

These things are all manageable – you just have to think about them in advance.

The following page offers the list of potential barriers you should consider.

▸ POTENTIAL BARRIERS YOU SHOULD CONSIDER ◂

#1 SOURCES OF JOY: do you look forward to your meals so much that they're significant sources of joy? I do. I love eating. I think about dinner all day. If so, how are you going to replace this? Knitting?

#2 FAMILY: families are difficult environments in which to lose weight. Everyone has advice, everyone has an opinion, they'll fill your fridge with stuff you don't want, they'll make demands on your time and emotional energy, and they don't usually like change. Families are a unit but a complicated one in which everyone has different goals. Not everyone will be on board with what you're doing at the same time that you are. I can't manage your family (I can hardly manage my own) but you will have to get them on board. Be nice. Be patient. Call a family meeting. It's easier when everyone's on board.

#3 TIME: following the advice in this book is likely to take more time than not following it. The advice works, but it's easier to order a takeaway. No one has infinite time and certainly not infinite energy. Don't embark on your diet by trying to prove this wrong.

#4 SOCIAL LIFE: if you're dating or socializing then sticking to a set of rules is harder. You may be less social for a while. Learn to make excuses.

#5 LOOKS, HEALTH, CONTROL: there's a strange phenomenon when people have weight-loss surgery and their weight changes rapidly: their chances of getting divorced seem to increase substantially. The reasons for this are hard to understand. I have spoken to surgeons about this complication of surgery and some of them suspect that the issue is the difficulty their partner has in adjusting to the new person. Many people find that they do literally become a different person when they lose large amounts of weight even if it happens slowly. People treat them differently and they feel different.

Simply being thinner won't fix as many of your problems as you'd like but the process of getting thinner involves a set of changes that will be hugely valuable across many areas of life. I suspect this is why the surgery can have more extreme consequences. The weight might just fall away but frequently the underlying problems that lead to the weight gain haven't been addressed.

THE PROGRAMME

What I learned while making the *How to Lose Weight Well* show is that everyone loves a plan. People need rules; I need rules; dogma works. The diet plans that worked for the participants in the shows were the ones that helped them join a kind of cult.

In a cult you don't have to make decisions for yourself and you can't question the rules. You just need blind obedience to the leader and total commitment to an overarching ideology. This model of leadership is great if you're trying to get people to live on your fortified ranch in Texas and prepare for the apocalypse, and it's great if you're trying to help people to lose weight. All the best-selling diets ask you to believe in a central idea. Sometimes it's an appealingly simple premise: carbs are toxic, or only eat what cavemen/women would have eaten. Other diets rely on a ludicrously complicated logic involving an analysis of your blood type or gut biome or the pH of the ash of the food in the diet... it doesn't really matter. Some religions are simple; some complex. The point is you have to be a believer.

All those diets have a deeply flawed scientific premise but they do pretty much work if you agree to stick to them. I just think you'll struggle because eventually everyone realizes that cavemen didn't live long and blood type just isn't that important.

I set out to empower the readers of this book but I've realized I don't always want to be empowered – I want to be told what to do.

So with that in mind here's the part of the book that caters to the fact that losing weight is tough and people need to have fewer decisions to make. I have made a four-step plan.

And I've made some meal plans so you don't have to think at all if you don't want to (see page 49). You can concentrate on your magically shrinking waist. Join my cult! It's the best one!

My cult, like any good cult (I imagine – I have never joined a cult), does have a guiding principle, which is to make sure that your daily calorie intake is less than or at least not greater than your calorie expenditure. Not a very exciting principle but a surprisingly controversial one.

A WORD ON CALORIES

Because calories are central to the logic of this diet I should explain what these mysterious things are. A calorie is a measurement of energy. To be exact, a calorie is the amount of energy required to raise the temperature of one litre of water by one degree Celsius (if you must know). So far so good? Well, no, things get confusing because, if you look on any packet of food in the UK at the calorie information, there are usually two kinds of calorie displayed: large calories, also known as kilocalories or kcal, and small calories or cal. The number you should care about is kcal. It will be the smaller of the two calorie numbers.

A FEW EXAMPLES:

A Tic Tac: 2 kcal
A jam doughnut: 200 kcal
A Big Mac: 563 kcal
A cabbage: 250 kcal
An apple: 55 kcal
An almond: 7 kcal
A 200g cod: 160 kcal
A 200g salmon: 340 kcal
A lamb chop with the fat left on: 240 kcal
A gram of fat: 9 kcal
A gram of carbohydrate: 4 kcal

If you set fire to a Tic Tac and used it to heat a saucepan with a litre of water in it, it would raise the temperature by about two degrees.

Now, we don't need to go back to your dreaded GCSE physics and chemistry lessons, but it is worth keeping in mind that your body needs energy to do everything from moving to thinking to keeping warm. Your body can get energy – calories – from three different kinds of nutrients: fat, protein and carbohydrates (which include sugars like glucose or dextrose, and starches). Your body has different processes to extract energy from each of these three kinds of molecule.

Because our caveman/cavewomen ancestors would have had to go without food for long periods of time (depending on the season and whether they got lucky hunting), we have evolved to store energy and enjoy eating calorific foods. When our food supply was sporadic, we needed to be able to eat more than a day's worth of calories in a single sitting so that we could survive a subsequent period of starvation. This is where our desire to eat more than we need comes from. It's not our fault. Blame cavepeople!

When you eat a meal, your body breaks down the protein, fat and carbohydrate molecules, uses what it needs and stores the rest. Some is stored in the form of a sugar called glycogen in the muscles and liver. The

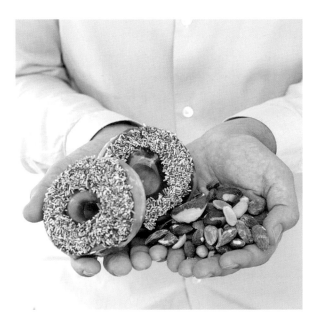

or sliced turkey you'll gain or lose weight exactly the same. The difference is that it's hard to eat large quantities of fat, protein or sugar on their own. Once they're combined they become far more delicious and it's extremely hard to stop eating them. If you don't believe me, fill a bowl with sugar and see how far you get eating it. But a mixture of cream and sugar? Well, that's basically ice cream. You can eat it till they wheel you away from the freezer.

Why don't we just count calories then? Isn't that the entire diet? Well, I strongly advise that you do keep an eye on the numbers of calories you're taking in and expending. But measuring your calorie intake and usage is pretty tricky. Any packet of food will claim to tell you both the calorie density (how many calories per 100g) and total calories. But it's very difficult to work out how many of the calories in a particular food will actually get into your body. You can set fire to different foods and see how much energy they release but since your body doesn't have a furnace in it, that doesn't give you a complete picture. After all, you could set fire to this book and it would probably release around 1,000 calories. If you ate it, though, it would release approximately zero calories to your body because it's made mainly of a kind of carbohydrate called cellulose, which you

rest is stored as fat. Sugar becomes fat; protein becomes fat; and fat becomes fat. So all you need to do is eat fewer calories than your body uses and it will turn to its fat reserves and start to mobilize them (usually by turning them into molecules called ketones, which make your breath smell rather bad but keep your brain working).

Why am I telling you all this? Well, there is quite a bit of debate about whether one calorie is the same as another. Will a calorie from sugar be more likely to make you gain weight than calories from fat or protein? There are many people who think so. I don't. I think if you ate 2,000 calories' worth of butter, sugar can't digest. Unless you're a goat. In which case you have the right digestive enzymes to break it down and turn it into sugar and so it will be making you fat rather than thin. This is the terrible irony of diet books for ruminants: they just eat them and get fat.

As well as this, it is very hard to know how many calories a person burns in a day as everyone is a little different: some people jitter and fiddle (the technical term for this is Non-Exercise Activity Thermogenesis or NEAT) more than others; people have different body compositions of different amounts of muscle and fat and so on. Even your smartphone/ fitness band isn't going to get it exactly right and could easily be out by a few hundred calories. It's worth noting that large differences in weight between people don't seem to be due to variations in 'metabolism'. Metabolism can roughly be thought of as how much energy your body uses at rest (the proper term is Basal Metabolic Rate or BMR).

But here's the bottom line. If you want to lose weight, you will have to use more calories than you consume and so even though it won't be exactly accurate you still need to know your numbers. It's boring but you'll need to weigh your portions, work out your daily calorie expenditure (I use myfitnesspal.com – I think it's good) and try to run a deficit. This book is about helping you do that. If it was easy as simply counting calories, I could stop writing now and go and have a drink and watch some TV. But that would make us both fat, so I'll continue.

THE FOUR STEPS TO LOSING WEIGHT WELL

STEP 1
IDENTIFY AND ELIMINATE YOUR ENEMIES

Who are your enemies? The legions of intelligent, hardworking people out there whose entire lives are devoted to making you eat more: the food merchants, the food scientists, the pub owners, the people in your office who seek personal validation by making everyone else eat their homemade lemon drizzle cake, your mother and anyone managing either a petrol station or a cinema (both these businesses rely almost entirely on selling you food to make a decent profit).

These people, and the foods they force upon you, are the enemy. You need to seek these fiends out and destroy or at least incapacitate them. You are at war with them. The old expression 'it takes two to tango' only applies if you are actually trying to tango. For just about everything else for which a tango is required to serve as a metaphor (usually some kind of fight) it only takes one. The other person just has to sit there. If you're passive in a war, you lose.

With this in mind I have compiled a set of rules that I try to live by.

▸ DR XAND'S RULES ◂

#1 EAT AS LITTLE PROCESSED FOOD AS POSSIBLE: you may be thinking that you already don't eat processed food. There are, after all, varying extremes of processing. There are microwave meals that have infinite shelf lives. By processed I really mean food that's had anything done to it.

> By definition, if anything has been done to food once it has been pulled out of the sea, off (or out of) an animal, or out of the ground – even if it has just been salted or peeled – it's been processed.

It's still worth thinking about two aspects of everything that goes onto your plate: how many things has it had done to it? And how many ingredients does it have? So here are the versions of this rule that seem reasonable to me.

▶ **Avoid foods that have had much done to them:** peel your own fruit, buy meat with bones in it, wash your own salad. You'll save money and you'll think more about what you're eating and the quantity you need. Try to cultivate an extreme hatred of food wrapped in plastic, made in a factory. Why? Because its job is to make you buy more of it, not to nourish you and fill you up. Now, if at this point you're thinking: "Yes, but I hate cooking/I have five children/I have three jobs/I don't have much money/all of the above", then don't despair. The recipes in this book are designed to make life as easy and cheap and fun as possible.

▶ **Buy food that has one ingredient:** the more ingredients it contains, the less you should buy. Why? The more ingredients the manufacturer adds, the easier it is to make you crave it. Think of the difference between salted and unsalted nuts (if you like nuts). If I buy a bag of unshelled, unsalted Brazil nuts (one ingredient) to eat, I'll have a satisfying snack, but if I buy a bag of dry roasted peanuts (about ten ingredients) or worse still those smoked almonds – also ten ingredients – which are like crack cocaine, I'll finish in a food coma. Those nuts aren't exactly more delicious, they're just harder to stop eating. You can find your own balance but every ingredient is added to make you eat more.

▶ **Avoid everything with MSG (or 'flavour enhancers'):** I'm not an MSG fascist. In fact I'd actively avoid a Chinese takeaway that says 'no MSG' because it will probably taste bland. MSG makes stuff taste amazing and I don't think it has half of the dismal effects that people claim it does. If you want proof of the power of MSG then have a party and make two bowls of just about anything: chilli, curry, pasta, guacamole, anything savoury. Add MSG to one and not the other. One bowl will remain full. The other will be seized by your guests as though they are auditioning for a part in a movie where the zombies finally feast. It's great stuff. But the danger is that it acts on your brain in a pretty fundamental way – it makes the food it's added to very hard to stop eating because it gives it that rich, irresistible umami flavour. It occurs naturally in products like Parmesan, mushrooms, anchovies and lots of fermented food.

Junk food is the food equivalent of pornography or slot machines or birthday cards for pets or mini-cab air-fresheners. I'm not opposed to those things *per se* but the world wouldn't be a worse place without them.

#2 DON'T EAT JUNK FOOD: this is similar to the rule about processed food, but it's stricter. My rule about processed food has to be a little flexible: I do buy salted nuts with the shells off. I do buy bacon. I'm not slaughtering chickens in my garden or making my own ketchup. Fair enough. But junk food is different. If you want to lose weight, you can't eat junk food.

What is junk food? It's food that is designed as entertainment. It's food that is made by a company with the aim not of feeding you but of briefly, temporarily and inadequately comforting you.

Since our early ancestors first learned to grow stuff and cook rather than just gathering and hunting, we have been able to choose our diets. There's nothing wrong with choice and a tasty meal. But a central idea about food seems to me that it should make you feel full, or at least satisfied. If you eat a piece of cheese and an apple an hour later, you'll feel less hungry than you would have if you hadn't eaten anything at all. This seems pretty straightforward, I hope. But if you eat a chocolate bar, packet of crisps, doughnut or any junk food, then an hour later you'll feel hungrier than if you'd eaten nothing. This is food that does the exact opposite of what it is supposed to. It's food that makes you hungry.

HERE'S HOW TO STOP EATING JUNK FOOD:

▶ **Remove it all from your house:** that means all packets of biscuits, chocolate bars and so on, go in the bin. It's no more of a waste to throw it away than to eat it. If you don't have junk food around, you can't eat junk food. This doesn't mean you can't snack while you lose weight, or that you have to be hungry. It just means you shouldn't eat stuff that will actually make you hungrier.

▶ **Identify the sources of temptation and change them if you can:** think about where and when you eat your junk food. I have friends who get it free at work in their fancy creative media jobs. I have other friends who only eat chocolate bars in the car on their commute. But mainly I have friends whose houses, because of their children or spouse, are filled with biscuits and snack bars. If it's there, you'll eat it. How do you make this work when not everyone in the house is trying to lose weight? It depends on who you are but it's not unreasonable to ask that it not be in the house, or at least not visibly. Other people can eat it elsewhere. If you live with an enthusiastic baker, then you will have to figure something out. A locked box is not too extreme.

▶ **Snack well:** I think there are a small number of snacks that work to lose weight. None of them are rice cakes or any other 'diet' food. My insight into this comes from a conversation I had with a man called Pavel Curtis at a conference at the Google headquarters in California. A software engineer and ferociously intelligent man, Pavel has spent his life solving complex problems for Microsoft and others. He said he realized one day that the main problem he had in his life was his weight and he felt strongly that someone as smart as him should be able to solve it. Accordingly he had made a spreadsheet of a vast number of foods and recorded (as I recall, over several months or even years) how well they satisfied his hunger. His conclusion was that, for him, the perfect

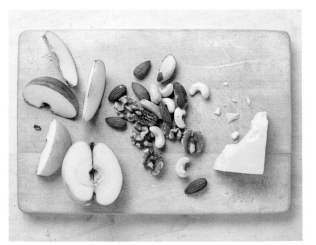

snack was an apple and either seven almonds or a 1-inch by 1-inch cube of cheese. He's a charismatic figure and I was young at the time and this made a great impression on me. I believe he's entirely right. You can experiment (he said that a pcar had worked better than an apple for his wife) but I'd say that your best bet is fresh fruit and or veg plus some fat and protein. 30g of cheese and an apple. Now, this is not your cue to keep a truckle of Cheddar on your work desk. But just about everywhere I go, I bring an apple or two and a handful of nuts. You can decant your day's snacks into a little bag at the beginning of the day and agree with yourself to only eat that and your meals. I'm lazy, poorly organized and forgetful (and frequently in America which is hell for anyone trying to avoid food), and even I can manage this.

#3 DON'T DRINK BOOZE

Alcohol for many people (including me) helps them socialize, date, network and relax. So why oh why am I saying don't drink? Well, there are two reasons.

Alcohol itself is high in calories – seven kcal per gram. The only thing that packs in more calories per gram is fat (nine kcal). A pint of ale is 200 kcal. That's the same as a doughnut. Lager isn't much better, around 180. A glass of wine (a large one in a pub) is about 150 kcal.

Kingsley Amis said that the point of a diet was to lose weight without reducing your alcohol consumption by a single drop.

If you pour it at home it's probably over 200. A bottle of wine is about 650 kcal. That's more than a Big Mac. I know that the newspapers run confusing stories about alcohol, so let me clear this up: drinkers do seem to live longer than teetotallers. However, I suspect (and I think the data backs me up pretty well on this) that those benefits are social rather than physical. Making friends, getting married, getting on at work are all good for life expectancy. The physical effects of alcohol aren't: it causes cancer, liver disease and heart disease.

The main problem with alcohol isn't that it's high in calories, though. If it was then you could just skip pudding or eat less at other meals. The problem is that it impairs your decision making both at the time, and for hours or (if you get hangovers like me) even days afterwards.

And once you've overdone it on Friday night, the rest of the weekend is a write-off. The effect of alcohol on your brain chemistry is profound and much of a hangover (the shaking, sweating and miserable paranoia)

> Being drunk, even a little merry, makes the takeaway more tempting, the slice of pizza harder to resist and the packet of pork scratchings (or whatever your weakness is — I appreciate not everyone is as enthusiastic as me about this particular delicacy) impossible to turn down.

seems to be related to changes in levels of particular neurotransmitters. With your brain chemistry all messed up, you need the full English breakfast to cope. And once you've had the full English, you've blown it for the day. You might as well put on a boxed set and recover with some popcorn and pizza. This, in many ways, is my ideal weekend. And I'm certainly not judging you if it's yours. You're welcome to do this every weekend. You're probably a great person to marry and spend time with. You are just not going to lose weight unless you stop doing it.

If you think you can manage to have a couple of pints a week, or a couple of glasses of wine and quit at that point and make sure you keep eating well then that's great. Keep drinking. But I can't. If I want to lose weight, I stop drinking completely. It's easy to turn down a drink if you say you're having a dry

month. It's hard if you say you'll just have one.

If you think you'll struggle to stop drinking (and especially if you start to get shaky or panicky without a drink) then see your doctor or seek some proper advice. It is possible to become physically dependent on alcohol and abrupt stopping can be dangerous.

Like every other aspect of losing weight, your relationship with alcohol should be deliberate and thoughtful.

#4 DON'T TAKE ANY PILLS OR VITAMINS: really, this is an easy rule to follow. Anything in a bottle or capsule that claims to have health benefits that isn't prescribed by a doctor (or at least advised by a naturopath you trust, if that's your thing) is not merely a waste of money; it's probably shortening your life. I think there are several good reasons to avoid all this stuff. Now I know the world is full of grumpy, sceptical people who don't believe in anything. They're dogmatic and closed-minded about all kinds of things like meditation, yoga, religion and cycling. I don't like those people and I'm not one of them. I have good reasons for spending some time discussing vitamin and mineral supplements and weight-loss pills.

Loads of people take this stuff. Even I have some lying around the house. My parents have cupboards full of fizzy vitamin C and

B12 tablets and my son takes multivitamin gummy bears every morning. Over 30% of adults in America take some kind of dietary supplement and we're not much different in the UK. The logic of taking vitamins goes something like this: years ago we used to have diseases caused by vitamin deficiencies. Sailors got scurvy because of lack of vitamin C on long sea voyages. Their teeth fell out and every day was a bad hair day and then they died from having severely weakened immune systems. Similarly, people got rickets from lack of vitamin D and had bone deformities. Because a lack of these substances caused bad hair, skin and bones, there is an appealing logic to the idea that an excess of these things will strengthen your hair/bones/immune system. This is no more true than the idea that, because your car doesn't run when it has no petrol in the tank, it will run better when

Linus Pauling won two Nobel prizes (in peace and chemistry) and he was a lifelong advocate of mega-doses of vitamin C. He was right about the structure of haemoglobin and about nuclear disarmament, but wrong about vitamin supplements. Two out of three isn't bad, I suppose.

the tank is full compared to half full, but it is the story with which vitamins are marketed. If you have a cupboard full of supplements, please don't feel gullible.

The lack of benefits of multivitamin and mineral supplements have been well studied. A study was published in 2013 in the *Annals of Internal Medicine* (a well-respected medical journal) reviewing a collection of trials of multivitamin supplements and single or paired vitamins that featured more than 400,000 participants. It found no clear evidence of a beneficial effect of supplements on all-cause mortality, cardiovascular disease or cancer. There are numerous other studies which support this finding and none which credibly undermine it. If you want to read more, this article is a good place to start: Guallar E, Stranges S, Mulrow C, Appel LJ, Miller ER. 'Enough Is Enough: Stop Wasting Money on Vitamin and Mineral Supplements' *Ann Intern Med.* 2013;159:850-851. The exception is vitamin D. Because we don't get much sunshine in the UK, deficiencies of this are very common and it's the one supplement you should consider taking. Other studies have found that certain ingredients (vitamin E, beta-carotene and high doses of vitamin A) may actually be harmful.

It's worth bearing in mind that the scientists doing this research would love to have found a benefit. This is a treatment which isn't just cheap; people actually pay for it themselves. Health ministries all over the world would be delighted to find that pills people are prepared to pay for out of their hard-earned and taxed income are reducing healthcare costs. But they aren't. We have searched high and low for benefits of supplements and found that, for the vast majority of people (adults), they are pointless.

Diet pills: these are also popular. Go into any high street healthfood shop or chemists and you will find a rack of diet pills. These are very bad news. There are only three ways a pill can make you lose weight.

▶ **If it makes you eat less:** but there is no pill available to do this. An appetite suppressant is one of the holy grails of modern pharmacology because it would make so much money for the company that invented it. I'd be first in line (unless there was a line for a hair tonic which they'd also invented, in which case I'd be in that line instead). I sincerely doubt that anyone will ever invent such a drug and here's why. Your brain's regulation of appetite is extremely important and it's a fundamental part of what allows us to exist. What we think of in modern life as the pursuit of pleasure (food and sex, for

example) is critical to survival. There are scientists working on mice and rats who have managed to invent drugs that reduce their appetites. But these drugs also mean they don't want sex or just about anything else. The desire and reward parts of our brains don't just focus on food: they are what motivate us to do just about everything important.

▶ **If it could make you absorb fewer of the calories that you eat:** there are lots of pills that claim to do this on the high street but only one of them has evidence to support its use. Its formal pharmaceutical name is Orlistat. You can get it over the counter in most chemists. It prevents your body from absorbing fat. It is obtainable by prescription on the NHS and is the only weight-loss pill currently approved by The National Institute for Health and Care Excellence (also known as NICE). This body sort of ensures high-quality treatment in the NHS. However, the side effects from not absorbing fat can be extremely unpleasant (including incontinence – I know from experience). This means that you will feel the bad effects of eating ice cream within a short time of eating it. Maybe it will work for you, but I personally find it more pleasant to pay a friend to smack me on the head with a rolled-up newspaper every time I reach for the chocolate.

▶ **If it could make you burn more of the calories you consume rather than storing them as fat:** there are drugs that claim to do this on the high street by increasing your metabolism. They are marketed as 'fat burners'. They almost always contain caffeine, garcinia cambogia or green tea extract. These pills do nothing for you that a cup of tea or coffee won't do. I'm a big fan of tea and coffee in all forms but no one ever changed their waistline significantly by drinking more tea, as you know if you've ever had a cup of tea. In fact, there are drugs that will alter your metabolism and literally burn your fat away but they are illegal and extremely dangerous.

I don't mean dangerous the way the doctors say everything is dangerous. I mean that you severely risk death. Changing your body's metabolism involves fiddling with some very important processes in your cells. I have interviewed both parents and doctors of people who have died taking drugs like this and the deaths are horrific and tragic. If you want to understand how profound the change in your body would have to be to burn off a significant amount of fat then simply go for a one-mile run. That will burn (depending on who you are and how much you weigh) about 100 calories. Which is very little. To take a drug that would make your body use more

calories than you ate, it would have to do something to you that was the equivalent of running while sitting still. Such drugs exist but they're profoundly dangerous.

In general, I'd say any food with a scientific claim that it will make you lose weight is nonsense. I can't produce good scientific evidence to support this statement but neither can the goji berry growers' marketing department.

"What about konjac root?" I hear you cry. OK I didn't hear you, but I'll tackle this anyway. This is a traditional Asian root the pulp of which is virtually indigestible. But it's safe to eat. So there we have it: a miracle product. No calories; safe to eat; fills you up. Except it doesn't work. Your body knows when it's getting tricked. Your brain isn't just happy to have a stomach full of stuff. If it was, you could just eat newspaper which is cheap and indigestible. Your brain is constantly monitoring the nutrients in your bloodstream so when you fill your belly with indigestible root fibre you won't feel like you've had a satisfying feed. You'll have a weird, confusingly full but empty feeling that will eventually make you go out and buy a tub of ice cream. And I wouldn't blame you. It's the wrong way of thinking about healthy eating. If you're hungry, then eat something healthy and call it a meal or a snack. Know how many calories are in it. If you're not hungry, then you're bored or anxious. Get a Rubik's cube.

#5 NO BLENDERS OR JUICES: the logic behind juicing and blending is similar to the logic behind taking vitamins. If a little of something is good for you then a lot of it will make you superhuman. So if you buy a blender, add enough green vegetables to feed a brachiosaurus for a week and then drink it down in one go, then this surely must be good for you? This seems not to be the case. The health benefits of eating fruit and vegetables are well documented: they provide essential nutrients and the fibre is good for your gut both in the short term (makes it easier to poo) and long term (seems to reduce your risk of cancer). The vegetables also fill you up and mean it'll be easier to eat fewer calories. The blender gets in the way of all these benefits. It chops up the fibre so it's not as good for your gut; it breaks up the plant cells meaning that the sugars are released quicker. So eating a blended orange or apple gives you sugar in about the same way as guzzling a fizzy drink.

There are so many books about why blending is great. They are all written by people who are either selling blenders or who love blenders for no good reason. Perhaps they are too lazy to chew but in any event they are not worth listening to. Also blenders are expensive. If you're blending your own stuff at home that's bad enough. If you're buying juice that's even worse. Just have a soft drink or a pint of beer. At least you won't be pretending it's doing you good. I don't care how much turmeric or ginger it has in it. The nutritional benefits of 'juice' are vastly outweighed by the sugar, the lack of fibre and the expense. It won't make you thin and it will make someone else rich. I could go on. Use your teeth. Chew up a plant. If it's broccoli, you can pretend that it's a tree and you're a giant. Anything other than blending and juicing please.

Chewing, which is an essential part of eating fruit and vegetables, is good for your breath (really the fibre scrubs off the dead cells from your tongue and teeth) and slows down your food consumption so that you don't eat as much. It also tastes nicer.

Should I tell people I'm on a diet? No. Say: "I don't eat junk food" or "I don't eat cake at the office. It makes me fat". This is true and it makes it hard for people to continue pestering you about it. It's also not fishing for a compliment. And you can say it whatever weight you are.

WORK: every workplace in the world offers temptation. The week you decide to change will be Free Brownie and Fried Chicken Week and there will be a birthday every day. And a drinks party every evening that you have to go to. Try to find a week to start changing which doesn't present too many of these obstacles – but they'll always be there. I make an unbreakable rule that I never, ever eat anything at the office that I didn't bring in. Birthdays, Christmas, whatever. I ignore it all. I don't see another way of doing it.

HOME: what about my family? If they aren't invested in you living long and feeling good then maybe you need to work on your relationship with them. Let's assume they are. The process of losing weight is uncomfortable for everyone because it involves changing some pretty fundamental routines. It is likely that you will be irritable and touchy. Be as nice as you can, and be patient when they're impatient with you. Easy for me to write. Maybe more reasonable advice would be: try not to murder all of them.

STEP 2
PREPARE TO
EAT WELL

GET YOUR PANTRY READY: oh, you don't live in Downton Abbey? Well then go through your kitchen cupboards. Remove all the junk and processed food. Give it away, or frankly, throw it away. Eating it is as much of a waste as not eating it. When you eat it, you become a human rubbish bin.

GET YOUR PHONE READY: download a calorie counting app, make a food diary in your calendar or notes section, and get an exercise app. The MyFitnessPal app will do all of this for you. And get a commitment app that will count your days of success. Or just use your phone to play Tetris every time you feel hungry. You can't eat while you play Tetris. Oh, and take a selfie. You'll see progress.

GET YOUR WORKPLACE READY: on Sunday, prepare and pack your snacks and lunch for the week. Or at least plan them exactly: where and what are you going to buy. Are there meetings, away days, out of office stuff or anything else you need to factor in? Are you going to arrive anywhere late or have to start very early?

SCHEDULE THE RIGHT START DATE: don't try to start the diet at the beginning of a three-week cruise with free drinks and a buffet with the captain every night. You'll ruin the holiday and lose no weight.

GET YOUR FAMILY READY: discuss your plan with your family. Work out how everyone's going to get fed at dinner time even if you're on a diet.

GET YOUR KITCHEN READY: losing weight well involves doing your own cooking. Many people dread this after a long day, but it should be a real pleasure. I know this sounds lame, like trying to persuade you that ironing is really 'me time', but cooking is pretty fun if you get set up right. There are a few bits of kit that turn cooking from a chore into a pleasure.

▶ **A kitchen TV, radio, audiobook or podcast:** anything to relax you and help you wind down while you cook. I watch reality cooking shows. It's nice not having Gordon Ramsay scream at me.

▶ There is one thing that is essential. Without one, life in the kitchen is misery; with one it's joy. **At least one good knife: sharp with a 6-inch or 8-inch blade:** you need to be able to get your knuckles around it and chop. It is very satisfying having this. It doesn't need to be very expensive: £20–40 will do nicely.

▶ **Please, oh please get a knife sharpener:** this is essential. Buy one when you buy your knife. Get it from the same company so that it works with that knife. There's no point in buying a £40 knife with the wrong sharpener. A dull knife makes everything harder and you will order takeaway.

▶ **A good chopping board:** this should fit in your sink so it's not a beast to clean. I like wood. It sounds nice and it looks nice. It won't blunt your knife.

▶ **A salad spinner:** no one ever has one of these and if you don't then your salad will be wet and disgusting. Buy a decent one. It makes eating lots of salad and veg easy.

▶ **A large serving bowl:** you can't eat enough greens if you can't serve them.

▶ **A large salad bowl:** you can't toss a salad in a tiny bowl. Get a nice big one. Bigger than you think.

▶ **A cast-iron skillet:** I know at this point I've lost some of you. I sound like some ludicrous hipster with a Victorian cookware fetish. But trust me. These pans are great. You can do everything in them and you don't have to be precious with them. They'll survive whatever abuse you throw at them.

▶ **A couple of heavy-bottomed non-stick saucepans:** get non-stick so cleaning them is easy. Get large ones so you can cook lots of veg.

That's it. You can cook just about every recipe in this book with this equipment. Georgie (who wrote the recipes) has made a complete list of everything you might need if you're feeling rich and ambitious (see page 55). I love to cook and her list is great. But you can get by with this short list almost every day.

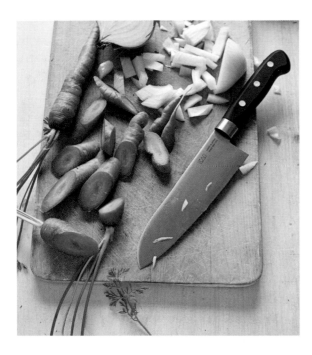

SHOPPING LISTS AND RULES: buy organic, cruelty-free meat if you possibly can and I try to buy organic vegetables and sustainable fish. I'm not very sentimental: I have eaten dog and guinea pig and I have kept both as pets (I didn't eat my pets). But I believe that good meat is good for you (for more on this, see page 108).

It is expensive to eat this way, and time and budget differ for everyone. Do what you can within your own limitations. If you have a local farmer's market, plus the inclination to buy your weekly ingredients from there, then that's brilliant. If your shopping routine involves buying everything from the supermarket, that's fine, too. Be organized and make detailed shopping lists: it will make your trip to the shops much more efficient and less painful.

STEP 3
EAT WELL

The basic premise of this diet is pretty simple. It is difficult to gain weight, or stay overweight, if you eat the right food. Most of what you put in your mouth should be green vegetables. OK they don't have to be green but most of them are: broccoli, kale, chard, spinach, lettuce and so on. If you know how to cook this stuff so that it's delicious (it's extremely easy), then giving up the other stuff won't seem nearly so wretched.

WHAT SHOULD BE ON YOUR PLATE?

VEGETABLES

I'm not interested in clean living and boredom and smiling through my salad while I pretend my life isn't falling to bits. I like gluttony, extravagance and fun. I like to see everyone leaving the table groaning and clutching their stomachs. I want to be able to tap my belly at the end of a meal and feel it's taut like a snare drum. But that doesn't mean I have to gain weight. I serve mountains of vegetables. Each dish is packed with fat, garlic, salt and whatever other flavours I'm in the mood for.

I can eat just about as much as I want. My main advice, I think, would be to have a go at a few of these recipes (see page 56). Make too much. Have a stuff up. See how they do as leftovers. Get stuck in.

I have a few reasons for advising you to eat lots of vegetables and they're all pretty simple.

▶ **Vegetables are good for you:** they're so good for you, I won't even bother assembling the medical research that supports this. They reduce your rates of just about every disease. They aren't magical, but they're close.

▶ **Vegetables slow you down:** you just can't eat a mountain of kale or broccoli fast unless you're the guy from that James Bond film with the metal teeth. You'll have to take your time, chew, enjoy and you'll have time to register when you're feeling full.

▶ **Vegetables speed you up (or at least keep you 'regular'):** modern diets and modern life mean that a vast number of people get constipated. It's hard to feel slim and happy when you've not had a poo for four days.

▶ **Vegetables fill you up:** but they contain, for their weight, relatively few calories. This seems obvious but it's the key reason to eat them when you're losing weight. It's virtually impossible to gain weight eating only vegetables. Now you'll have to add a few calories to make them interesting and tasty but unless you batter and deep-fry them, it's hard to really mess this up.

▶ PRO-TIPS ON EATING VEGETABLES ◀

Making it taste good isn't difficult. It can be as simple as this:

▶ **Buy a pile of green stuff:** it really doesn't matter what: kale – broccoli, spinach, Swiss chard, dandelion greens. Even radish tops, beetroot leaves and carrot tops: you can just eat them instead of putting them in the rubbish bin. If it's leaves and it's in a supermarket you can eat it.

▶ **Heat some oil in a pan:** get it nice and hot. Almost smoking. Chuck in the leaves. They'll sizzle. Stir until they wilt. Salt heavily and/or add a splash of soy sauce or miso dressing or lemon juice. Tip into a bowl. Eat.

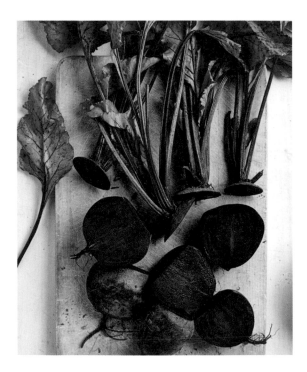

▶ **I've left out some of the hassle – you'll have to wash and chop stuff – but basically it's that easy:** a head of broccoli isn't for a family of four. It's for you! All of it! A bag of kale doesn't serve a dinner party. It serves you. Want to add flavour? Smash some cloves of garlic with the flat of your knife. Don't even peel the garlic, you can eat the peel and your hand won't smell afterwards. Fry the garlic until it's going a little brown on the edges. Throw in a bunch of dried chilli flakes if you like it spicy. It is virtually impossible to mess this up though you'll need to do it a couple of times so that you get a feel for when it's ready. It takes under five minutes, it's cheap, and you only have one pan to wash.

PROTEIN

Your stomach isn't like a petrol tank that clicks off when it's full of vegetables. Your brain is constantly measuring what's entering your bloodstream – fat, sugar, protein – and if it's not getting enough it'll be sending out signals that it wants more. So, while it's hard to gain weight eating only vegetables, it's also hard to eat only vegetables. Your brain will keep demanding cheeseburgers. And there's always room for cheeseburgers. And ice cream. So you do need other things as well.

Protein fills you up and makes you feel satisfied. And it's tasty. Once you've got a heaping pile of vegetables on your plate all you need to go with it is a nice piece of protein and you're done. It is so easy to cook this stuff it blows the mind. Take a steak, a pork chop, a piece of salmon. Salt both sides. Stick it in a frying pan on high heat. Turn it halfway through. Serve with whatever condiment or dressing you want. Or roast a chicken. You don't need to take off the skin or cut off the fat. Just cook it and put it on the plate by the vegetables.

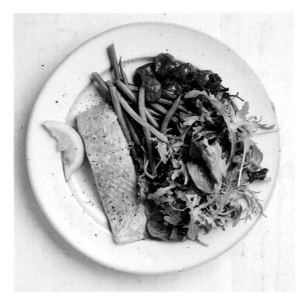

FAT

Fat makes you feel good. You need fat for your body to function. And it doesn't do you harm in the ways that are commonly believed. This is not a low-fat diet. You do need to be a little wary of the sheer density of calories in fat: a tablespoon of olive oil is over a hundred kcal. But fat doesn't stimulate your body to release insulin (see Carbs, over the page) and it doesn't make you crave more. I spent a month eating an incredibly high-fat diet with zero carbs: so I ate almost exclusively cheese and fatty cuts of meat. I didn't even have vegetables. It was delicious and I never felt hungry. But I did get bored and eventually stopped eating that way.

CARBS

Unless you've been living in a cave for the last decade (and if you have, I doubt you need to lose any weight) then you're aware of the idea of low-carb diets. The logic goes something like this: sugar and carbohydrates (which you can think of as kinds of sugar, since starch is just lots of joined-up sugar molecules in a chain) make your body release a hormone called insulin. Insulin reduces your blood sugar by allowing the sugar to enter cells. Insulin is extremely closely related to Growth Hormone (it's just called: growth hormone), which does what it says on the tin and makes you grow, and insulin does seem to make people grow in the same way. So there is an idea that if you eat food that makes you release a lot of insulin then the insulin will make you fat. I think this is baloney.

You gain weight if you eat too many calories. Low-carb diets stop you eating too many calories. If you take the bread and beans and ketchup out of a fried breakfast, it's a pretty healthy meal.

The reason to reduce your carb intake is that it's really easy to eat far too much. All nations and cultures have some traditional carbs but in the UK we also have a tradition of just eating a tonne of carbs. We'll have garlic bread as a side dish to a bowl of pasta. We cover cake in custard. It makes me proud to be British. But it also makes me fat.

HOW TO MAKE STUFF TASTE NICE

In my first year as a doctor, I was excused from a ward round because I smelled too strongly of garlic. The night before I had had dinner with my mother and I had eaten a roasted bulb of the stuff. It looked like a half grapefruit: the top had been cut off, exposing all the cloves like segments. It had been drizzled with olive oil and salt and then roasted until it was golden brown and sticky and delicious. Garlic was oozing out of my every pore the next morning and my consultant, a lovely man called Dr Darowski, just smiled indulgently and told me that this was not an acceptable way to appear in front of people who were sick enough to be in hospital. I spent the day doing other odd jobs that didn't involve patient care and not breathing on anyone. Sometimes compromises have to be made.

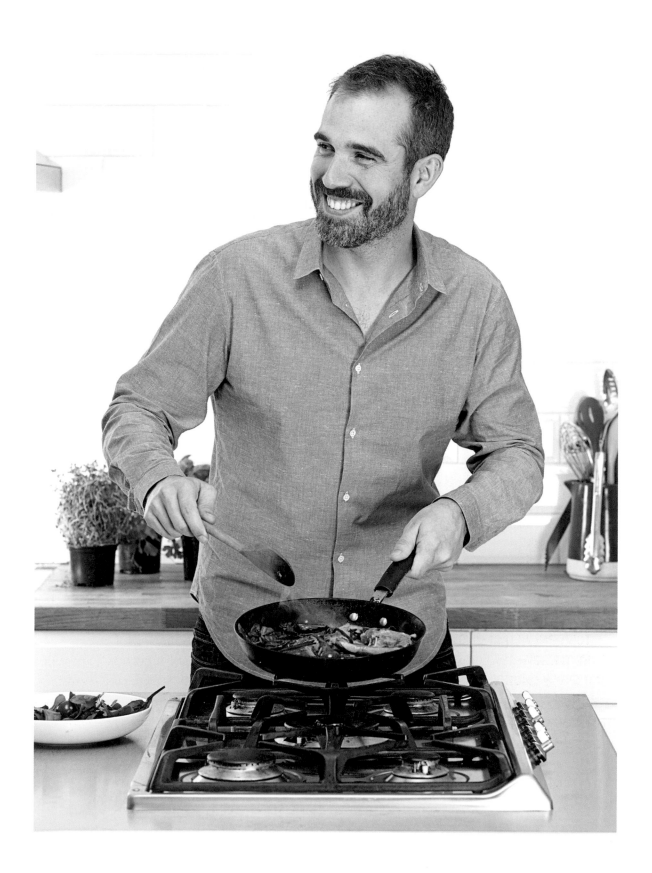

Since I'm not advocating a low-fat diet, making sure the food you eat tastes nice is pretty easy. Your cuts of meat can be juicy and your greens drizzled with olive oil or accompanied by a knob of butter.

In general, if something tastes bland, the cause is that there's not enough salt or fat. These two ingredients have been unfairly demonized. While it is true that salt does contribute to high blood pressure, it makes far less difference than being overweight. The studies on salt-restricted diets to reduce people's blood pressure also find that removing enough salt to make a difference makes food virtually inedible. If you have high blood pressure then discuss this with your GP but for the majority of people I don't think good sea salt in home-cooked vegetables is the enemy. Salt (or sodium) in processed food, on the other hand, is the enemy.

Georgie (pictured here with me) and I have had great conversations about flavour. She likes everything I like but she's more precise and more inventive. The recipes in this book are exactly what I cook at home... but even better and incredibly easy.

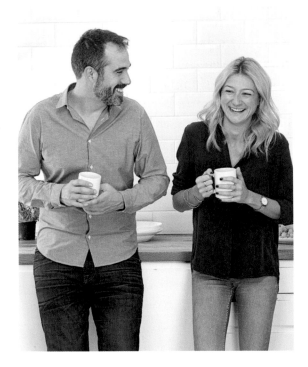

SNACKING

We're terrible at snacking in the UK. Snacks are a useful part of a healthy diet. My main advice on snacking is this: do it when you're hungry, not when you're bored. Plan and measure out your snacks in advance (the night before). Make them yourself: an apple and a piece of cheese; a handful of nuts and a pear (see page 27). I aim for high-fat, high-protein, low-carb snacks. Know how many calories are in them (I suggest about 200–250). Choose the time window in which you'll eat them (maybe 11AM and 3:30PM depending on your life). Get a routine for these that will help you fight off hunger but allow you to stop. When you're bored, drink green tea or black coffee, or chew gum or something else with no calories in it.

WHAT TO DO ABOUT PUDDING?

There are desserts in this book. Life without pudding is no life at all. But as I've suggested, there are kinds of pudding that are toxic and that you won't be able to stop eating. My rule would be: make your own pudding, and it should be fruit-centric at least six nights per week. You can eat all the oranges, grapefruit and apples you want. They're fun to peel while you watch TV or chat and they won't make you gain weight. My particular favourites are grapefruits. I chill them and then chop them up with a very sharp knife into a huge pile and eat them with cold juice running down my chin. With just about everything other than fruit it's worth considering the number of calories very carefully.

STEP 4
LIVE WELL

Most diet books are like 'teach yourself the guitar' books. I have bought a few of these, and a guitar, and yet I cannot play a note. I had the determination and commitment needed to buy a book and an instrument. What I have so far failed to do is alter my life in a way that allows me to learn the guitar. I blame the books for this. None of my guitar books (OK, I bought several) ever said quite how much dedication and practice and frustration and disappointment is involved in learning an instrument in your mid-thirties (OK, late-thirties). They just said "follow these ten easy steps". They didn't mention that I'd need hours of time that I don't have, and quantities of confidence and self-belief that I think are reserved for professional politicians, MMA fighters and gameshow hosts.

Losing weight well is even harder than learning the guitar and, while this book does contain rules and advice, I think you could ignore most of it if you understand one important thing: if you want to lose weight and maintain that weight loss you will have to change your life.

What we eat is intimately linked to every single part of our lives. What we eat is determined by the lives we choose or are forced to live. It's determined by the places and ways that we have to shop, by our jobs, our families, our friends and our ambitions and the patterns of our thoughts. I don't mean you'll have to change things in a bad or dramatic way but you cannot change what is on your plate (or in your mouth) without altering the world around you. This is cause for optimism not pessimism.

Everyone gains weight because they consume more calories than they need to get through the day, but this is an utterly unhelpful analysis of the problem (see page 20 if you don't know what a calorie is). You're not in a position where you want to lose weight simply because you overeat. We have to ask why we're eating more than we need. Everyone will have different reasons and so each person's trick to losing weight well will be a little different.

Other diet books — almost all of them — are one-size-fits all. This one is different.

That's why this isn't simply a book of rules and low-calorie recipes that will make you feel full and be reasonably easy to cook. For a 'diet' to work, it can't just be a food plan, it has to be a way of life. *Eye-roll.* Look, I don't want you to chant or meditate or only wear clothes that are the colours of the sunrise. I just mean identify the behaviours and practices that will help you eat well. I hope that the three steps preceding this one help you do this. 'Live well' is the final step and if you get this right the rest will follow, I'm sure.

EXERCISE

If you want an example of how a little exercise allows you to diet less, then look no further than professional cyclists. I spent some time talking with the nutritionist for the Sky Sports cycling team. It's his job to fuel the riders during training and during the Tour de France. He was fascinating about the starvation they endure. The cyclists really don't want to be carrying a single extra gram up the hills and so they starve themselves thin. These are athletes who are burning thousands of calories a day on their bikes and they're all dieting to get ready for race season.

The point is, it's extremely difficult to lose weight by exercising unless you change what you eat. It's almost impossible, in fact,

unless you're a cycle courier (in which case I would really love to hear from you about why you bought this book) or a polar explorer (in which case you should fatten up for your next trip). Exercise is an appetite stimulant and it also makes us artificially believe we've earned a doughnut. In reality, a single doughnut is about 30 minutes of hard exercise. And no one ever has a single doughnut.

WHY DO EXERCISE IF IT DOESN'T HELP YOU LOSE WEIGHT?

▶ **It's a reason to lose weight:** you'll get better at it the more you lose.

▶ **It's very good for you:** the Academy of Medical Royal Colleges said in a recent report entitled 'Exercise: the Miracle Cure' that if physical activity was a drug, it would be classed as a wonder drug.

▶ **If you're losing weight, I don't want you to lose muscle:** I want you to lose fat. It's great to have lots of muscle even if it weighs a lot. Muscle makes you healthy.

▶ **It will make you look better:** losing fat isn't much good without building muscle.

▶ **It will make you function better:** late nights, carrying babies, just being alive will be easier if you're in good shape.

▶ **It will make you feel better:** your aches and pains will improve.

▶ **It will allow you to measure progress:** the scales will help but you'll notice how far you can walk and how much easier it is to get upstairs or run a mile.

▶ **For all the above reasons:** it reflects your motivation – i.e. a respect for your body and yourself.

▶ **Exercise is deeply personal:** I like walking my dog, cold water swimming, doing chin-ups and press-ups. Other people love yoga; I love recommending yoga.

MY SUGGESTIONS

▶ **Do exercises that use your own body weight:** press-ups, sit-ups, pull-ups. If you don't know how to do these or you can't do a single pull-up or press-up then start very slowly. Google 'push-ups for complete beginners'. I know this seems lazy of me, but a video is far more useful than a page of prose for this kind of thing.

▶ **Buy trainers, sports clothes and a chin-up bar:** use the money you save from not joining a gym.

▶ **Do something rather than nothing:** ten push-ups is only ten times more than one. But one push-up is infinitely more than none. So set the bar low. I don't want you to dread this.

▶ **Aim for ten push-ups, ten sit-ups and ten pull-ups per day for a month:** set reminders on your phone. If you can't do a push-up, kneel to do them. If you can't do a pull-up, then stand on a chair and use your legs a little until you can.

▶ **Aim to walk for 40 minutes, three times per week, for a month:** if that doesn't fit with your schedule, do 20 minutes. Don't do none.

▶ **If you have the money, the aptitude and the time, then buy a decent bike:** buy the stupid padded shorts. Cycle everywhere. This is probably the only thing that is likely to impact your weight (I know I said Sir Bradley Wiggins still had to diet but he's trying to cycle up mountains – it's different). In the summer when I use my bike every day, I think I am expending about 1,500 calories more than normal. Provided I eat good food, it's hard to gain weight when I'm doing that.

TIDY UP

I do mean tidy your house. It is extremely difficult to feel happy amid clutter and dirt and disorganization and feeling happy is important to losing weight. It's also very difficult to cook, store food well and most of all to feel disciplined when your house is preventing you doing those things and announcing to the world, and much more importantly to you, that you aren't disciplined in any way. I don't just mean wipe down the surfaces. I mean throw away your old clothes, books you haven't read, old magazines. Whatever the charity shop will take, let them take it. It can clutter someone else's life up. There are many books on tidying. My favourite is *The Life-Changing Magic of Tidying Up* by Marie Kondo.

Perhaps you're living in spotless perfection with no clutter and no junk and you're rolling your eyes at me and thinking that it hasn't helped you lose weight. But even if that's the case – and it isn't for most people – you still need to tidy your life. This change is going to be significant and many of your relationships need tidying up. I once spent an extremely happy weekend with a family (mum, dad and two teenage daughters) trying to make them healthier as a family. They tidied and cleaned their house. But they also adjusted who shopped, who cooked and how they would support each other. They were one of the nicest families I've ever met (I made a TV show about them) and I was very nervous about disrupting a happy home and somehow sterilizing it. After all, some of what makes a family a family is the clutter and shared memories and well-understood relationships and roles. But we did it. Their house still feels like a home but they lost weight (a lot of weight), kept it off and will live longer and more happily as a result. I wish I could write a formula for doing this, and I have tried. But everyone's family and social world are different. The best tools you have are love and common sense. Try to prioritize these. Do one thing that symbolically says – I can achieve something. I can get stuff done.

> Of course, it's not about tidying your house; it's about tidying your life.

In order to lose weight well, you will need to arrive at a moment when you decide you want to change; when you permanently alter the way in which you approach this problem. For some people this involves hitting 'rock bottom'. I can relate to this. By the time I decided I should lose some weight my blood pressure was skyrocketing and my blood sugar was well on the way towards diabetes. The decision for me was instantaneous (I remember thinking "this is absurd, I am going to change" and not really looking back). For other people it is more gradual.

This book aims to push you towards that decision point and to give you the tools you need to take advantage of it. You'll need to make a plan, you might need to buy a set of scales or some kitchen equipment. All of the preparation is detailed in this book. But at some point you're ready to set a day and begin and not look back.

There will be setbacks and difficult days but I'd prefer you didn't think of it as falling off the wagon. I'd prefer that you stepped off the wagon, had a break, deliberately had a day or two where you didn't try to run a calorie deficit, and then got back on the wagon again. I'm not trying to sign you up to a lifetime of no booze and no ice cream. But I think you should be deliberate about your choices around those things.

So that's the plan: change your life.

MEAL PLANS

There are three plans. They're all pretty similar, they all use the recipes in this book. I personally use all of them depending on how my life looks on any given week. They are based on how many meals you need to eat in a day. Only you can judge this and it will vary from day to day.

HOW TO START YOUR DIET AND CHOOSE YOUR MEAL PLAN

▶ On the first week, stick to the number of meals that you usually have each day. This diet emphasizes cooking and taking control by counting calories and by eating freshly cooked food. You'll need to get used to preparing and eating more vegetables and shopping differently.

▶ Keep a food diary and at the end of the week evaluate how you feel based on what you've eaten. Did you feel good every day? Which meal did you enjoy the most? Which did you most look forward to?

▶ Losing weight will involve figuring out where you need to cut calories. Personally, I find most days that it's easiest to stay hungry until dinner. Other people can't stand this so work towards a solution for you.

A WORD ON FASTING

Fasting – in terms of dieting – doesn't mean not eating. It's properly called 'intermittent fasting' and it means going without food for between 14 and 24 hours. Fasting is something that people will give you a hard time for in my experience. When I announce that I haven't had breakfast, I get a barrage of grumbling from my colleagues about how this behaviour is not merely fattening but profoundly immoral and irresponsible. It is as if they are in the pay of the breakfast cereal lobby. I have used various rebuttals over the years. "There is a professor of nutrition at the Harvard School of Public Health who only eats one meal per day!", I say (his name is Dr David Ludwig should you wish to cite him in similar arguments). I have also invoked my six years at Oxford and my master's degree in public health from Harvard, along with the large amount of medical evidence, that fasting is safe and an effective way of losing weight. This all falls on deaf ears and makes me sound like a know-it-all. In the end it's easier to lie and say you had the full English.

The scientific research on fasting makes compelling reading (OK, it's not the new Dan Brown or Gillian Flynn but I enjoyed it!): it does seem that you can lose weight by fasting even if you don't reduce your overall weekly calorie intake. The way in which this works isn't clear but some researchers describe fasting as being a good kind of stress on your body, like exercise, and that it promotes fat burning. There is one problem with the fasting data though: it isn't for everyone. If you start 100 people on a fasting diet like the 5:2, you'll find that six months later the majority of them have quit. Those that have stuck to it tend to do well. But most people don't find it suits them.

My advice is to try it and bear the following things in mind. Your body has memory of the way you used to eat. If you have a chocolate bar at 10AM one day, the next day at 10AM your body will expect a chocolate bar. Fasting can therefore be a shock to the system and the first day you're likely to feel hungry. It does get better. My way of dealing with hunger is to remember that feeling hungry isn't too bad and it is possible to function quite well when you're hungry. After all, our poor caveman/woman ancestors had to get stuff done (cave painting, mammoth slaying, wheel inventing, etc.) and they were hungry much of the time. And I also try to remember that if I have a big lunch, I go into a food coma until 5PM.

Fasting doesn't have to come with a safety warning but it is worth remembering that there is good evidence that we do function less well when we're hungry. You function less well when you're full, tired, worried and all sorts of other brain states but it is undeniable that after a long fast (say 24 hours) you're less competent to operate heavy machinery than if you hadn't fasted.

My personal experience is that fasting works well much of the time. I have a nine-to-five job for quite a bit of the time in which I teach and do research. I start the day with a cup or two of black coffee and then eat all my calories in the evening in a big, tasty meal. I don't have to exercise much restraint on that meal and I finish it feeling full and happy. When I'm trying to lose weight, I'm going to have to be hungry some of the time, so I'd rather spend the day thinking about a hearty dinner and not wondering why I'm hungry.

The amount of hunger you can cope with depends for many people on knowing how long it's going to last and what will happen at the end of it. It's like being sleep deprived. If you're tired on holiday it's no big deal; the same amount of tiredness on a Monday morning prior to a busy week is almost impossible to cope with. Similarly, I can cope with having one meal a day to look forward to most of the time. But when I'm working away from home, in places where the evening meal is going to be dismal or possibly non-existent, this means that there isn't much to look forward to at the end of a period of hunger. At these times I tend to have three meals per day.

MEAL PLAN (A)
3 MEALS A DAY

Eating three good-quality meals per day means you won't have any episodes of severe hunger. And if you do, you can manage them by snacking. But you'll have to be careful about counting your calories and you won't be able to have a real stuff up for any of the meals. But that can be good for lots of people. Preventing indigestion and learning portion control for many is far more important than enjoying one big meal per day.

DAY BY DAY

MONDAY
Breakfast: Perfect Porridge (page 178)
Lunch: cheese and a dressed salad
Dinner: Steak and Garlicky Green Veg (page 68).

TUESDAY
Breakfast: Bacon & Eggs (page 176)
Lunch: leftover dinner from last night. Make sure to weigh it.
Dinner: Asian Red Cabbage, Carrot & Spinach Slaw (page 62) with Five-Spiced Beef in Little Gem (page 112)

WEDNESDAY
Breakfast: Granola (page 180)
Lunch: leftover dinner from last night. Make sure to weigh it.
Dinner: Japanese Rice & Tuna Bowl (see page 134)

THURSDAY
Breakfast: Breakfast Scramble (page 182)
Lunch: cheese and a dressed salad
Dinner: Turmeric Tandoori Chicken Thighs (page 100) with Chicory, Orange & Walnut Salad (page 72)

FRIDAY
Breakfast: Spinach Masala Omelette (page 186)
Lunch: leftover dinner from last night. Make sure you weigh it.
Dinner: Fish Pie with Pea & Parsnip Mash (page 130) and Avocado, Fennel & Asparagus Salad (page 64)

SATURDAY
Breakfast: Sweet Potato Pancakes (page 184)
Lunch: leftover dinner from last night. Make sure you weigh it.
Dinner: Kale, Avocado & Soft Egg Salad (page 154)

SUNDAY
Breakfast: Sweet Potato Pancakes (page 184)
Lunch: cheese and a dressed salad
Dinner: Pork & Fennel Seed Meatballs with Cavolo Nero (page 102)

MEAL PLAN (B) 2 MEALS A DAY

I have two meals per day about half the days of the year. I don't wake up hungry (possibly because I had a pretty big evening meal) but a light, late lunch prevents me getting too slow in the afternoon and I can commute home feeling a little hungry but knowing that I can still have a pretty decent dinner.

DAY BY DAY

MONDAY

Breakfast: Black coffee or tea, or other calorie-free drink
Lunch: cheese and a dressed salad
Dinner: Steak and Garlicky Green Veg (page 68). GO FOR IT.

TUESDAY

Breakfast: Black coffee or tea, or other calorie-free drink
Lunch: handful of nuts and 2 pieces of fruit
Dinner: INDULGE. Asian Red Cabbage, Carrot & Spinach Slaw (page 62) with Five-Spiced Beef in Little Gem (page 112)

WEDNESDAY

Breakfast: Black coffee or tea, or other calorie-free drink
Lunch: leftover dinner from last night. Make sure you weigh it.
Dinner: Japanese Rice & Tuna Bowl (see page 134). BRING IT.

THURSDAY

Breakfast: Black coffee or tea, or other calorie-free drink
Lunch: cheese and a dressed salad
Dinner: Turmeric Tandoori Chicken Thighs (page 100) with Chicory, Orange & Walnut Salad (page 72). Because you earned it.

FRIDAY

Breakfast: You're getting the idea, right? Black coffee or tea, or other calorie-free drink
Lunch: leftover dinner from last night. Make sure you weigh it.
Dinner: Fish Pie with Pea & Parsnip Mash (page 130) and Avocado, Fennel & Asparagus Salad (page 64)

SATURDAY

Breakfast: Still black coffee or tea, or other calorie-free drink
Lunch: leftover dinner from last night. Make sure you weigh it.
Dinner: Kale, Avocado & Soft Egg Salad (page 154)

SUNDAY

Breakfast: Pancakes. It's Sunday. Enjoy!
Lunch: keep digesting those pancakes
Dinner: Pork & Fennel Seed Meatballs with Cavolo Nero (page 102)

MEAL PLAN (C)
1 MEAL A DAY

It can take getting used to. You'll be hungry and maybe a little slow for some of the afternoon, although since you'll have roughly 22 hours between meals, depending on how slowly you eat, this way of eating probably does get you towards the effects of fasting on burning fat so that you may get an extra benefit. You might struggle with discipline, especially if you shop on your way home when you're hungry (this can get expensive). But it's really hard to gain weight on one meal per day. You can manage it if you eat pizza and ice cream but if you stick to our recipes or variations on them then you'll be fine.

DAY BY DAY

MONDAY
Breakfast: Black coffee or tea, or other calorie-free drink
Lunch: nope!
Dinner: You can feast. Steak and Garlicky Green Veg (page 68).

TUESDAY
Breakfast: Black coffee or tea, or other calorie-free drink
Lunch: zip
Dinner: YUM. Asian Red Cabbage, Carrot & Spinach Slaw (page 62) with Five-Spiced Beef in Little Gem (page 112)

WEDNESDAY
Breakfast: Still black coffee or tea, or other calorie-free drink
Lunch: nada
Dinner: Japanese Rice & Tuna Bowl (see page 134). YES!

THURSDAY
Breakfast: Black coffee or tea, or other calorie-free drink
Lunch: you're getting the idea by now I bet. A big plate of nothing.
Dinner: Turmeric Tandoori Chicken Thighs (page 100) with Chicory, Orange & Walnut Salad (page 72). NICE.

FRIDAY
Breakfast: Same old black coffee or tea, or other calorie-free drink
Lunch: not today, thanks
Dinner: glorious Fish Pie with Pea & Parsnip Mash (page 130) and Avocado, Fennel & Asparagus Salad (page 64)

SATURDAY
Breakfast: Sweet Potato Pancakes (page 184) – why not? You did well all week.
Lunch: have a long walk
Dinner: Kale, Avocado & Soft Egg Salad (page 154). OH YES.

SUNDAY
Breakfast: Black coffee or tea, or other calorie-free drink
Lunch: Take a walk, prepare dinner and the coming week's meals
Dinner: Slow-Roast Shoulder of Pork (page 106). Crunch the crackling. Enjoy.

RECIPES & COOKING

CHECKLIST FOR GETTING STARTED

▶ You need a way of tracking what you eat and your progress: a diary, a calendar or a notes app on your phone work well.

▶ Measure your waist circumference. It's a better indicator of health than weight. Check in once per week.

▶ Get some decent digital scales. Weigh yourself every day.

▶ Calculate how many calories you need per day. Search for 'total daily energy expenditure calculator' online. It's very easy.

▶ Plan and record your exercise regimen in your diary/calendar/MyFitnessPal. I'd start with a 30-minute walk three times per week and some strength work (see Step 4 on page 44) on the other days.

▶ Install a calorie counter app on your phone so that you can work out how much is in your meals easily. I use MyFitnessPal.

▶ Write your meal plans for the first two weeks.

▶ Write down the big obstacles for the first two weeks (is there a wedding or a work event?)

EVERY DAY

▶ Do weigh yourself in the morning and record the weight and the time.

▶ Do write down every meal and the calories in the meals.

▶ Do some exercise.

▶ Do not worry about what happened yesterday.

▶ Do not panic about what your scales say.

THE FIRST FEW DAYS

▶ **The weight may fall off.** There's less food hanging around in your gut and less sugar holding water in your muscles and liver. This rate of weight loss is very unlikely to continue.

▶ **The weight may not fall off.** Small reductions in body fat are completely masked by the fluids we drink. If you eat a salty meal, you'll retain water and gain several kilos.

▶ **Either way don't panic.** Keep an eye on the calories and keep writing down your weight. You will get there.

▶ **If you eat badly in the morning, you'll write off the rest of the day.** This seems to be nearly universal. Recommit every day, and avoid the self-loathing.

When I began searching for a professional cook with whom to collaborate on the recipes in this book, I was looking for someone who cared about making delicious food quickly and easily with normal affordable ingredients.

I wanted recipes that would make healthy food accessible for everyone. I didn't want to obsess over sugar or carbs, or fat if possible. Georgie is the perfect partner in all these respects: she's an awesome cook and happy to make a recipe reasonable for people with busy lives. Sure, a 72-hour veal stock might improve the dish. But a cube will do. The recipes in here are delicious and are exactly the kinds of food that I eat every day to maintain my weight or, when I need to, lose some.

A WORD ON NUTRITIONAL INFORMATION

All the nutritional information given for each recipe in the following pages (fat, protein, sugar, fibre and calories) is per serving.

USEFUL KITCHEN EQUIPMENT

This is Georgie's list and a more complete one than I suggested earlier on page 35. It depends on how rich you're feeling and how much you love cooking:

- ▶ Sharp knives and sharpener
- ▶ Scissors
- ▶ Ladle
- ▶ Potato masher
- ▶ Vegetable peeler
- ▶ Whisk
- ▶ Chopping boards
- ▶ Non-stick saucepans and frying pans
- ▶ Baking tray and ovenproof ceramic dishes
- ▶ Colander and sieve
- ▶ Grater
- ▶ Mixing bowls
- ▶ Wooden spoons and spatula
- ▶ Kitchen scales
- ▶ Food processor: this is Georgie's top recommendation.

VEGETABLE SIDES

This is the most important section of the book for weight loss. You can eat tonnes of all this stuff. The more you eat, the fuller you will get and the less need you will have for a doughnut or that glass of wine.

DRESSINGS

Of all the things I learned from Georgie, the most rewarding is that drizzling a delicious dressing on to the simplest plate of vegetables can elevate it into something wonderful. Here are six of my favourite dressings: try them and find your favourites to make again and again. They all keep well in the fridge for a week. Try stirring them through soups, salads and vegetable dishes, or sprinkle over meat and fish.

All of these are suitable for 2 servings of salad.

For all the dressings (except the Avocado), simply whisk the ingredients together with a fork, or shake together in a jam jar (with the lid on).

SIMPLE LEMON DRESSING

6 tbsp olive oil
juice of 1 lemon
good pinch of salt

DIJON DRESSING

6 tbsp olive oil
1 tbsp cider vinegar
½ garlic clove, finely chopped
pinch of salt
1 tsp Dijon mustard
1 tsp honey

GREEN DRESSING

6 tbsp olive oil
1 tbsp cider vinegar
juice of ½ lemon
1 heaped tbsp chopped herb leaves (I like flat-leaf parsley, coriander or dill, or a combination)
pinch of salt
½ garlic clove, finely chopped

MISO & SESAME DRESSING

This also makes a wonderful sauce in which to stir-fry meat or vegetables.

1 heaped tsp miso paste
2 tbsp sesame oil
2 tbsp olive oil
juice of 1 lemon

TAHINI DRESSING

2 tsp tahini
juice of ½ lemon
6 tbsp olive oil
2 tbsp water
pinch of salt
1 tsp honey

AVOCADO DRESSING

¼ avocado, peeled and stoned
7 tbsp olive oil
pinch of salt
¼ garlic clove
juice of 1 lemon

Put all the ingredients into a food processor or blender and process until smooth.

FAT (G): 7.2
PROTEIN (G): 2.2
SUGAR (G): 4.5
FIBRE (G): 4.2
KCAL: 154
SERVES: 2

A simple but substantial side dish; use in place of potatoes for a filling but nutritious alternative. Next time, try whizzing the cooked squash and dressing together in a food processor, or just mashing the old-fashioned way, for an interesting mash.

ROAST SQUASH WITH CHILLI & CORIANDER

½ butternut squash
1 tbsp olive oil, plus more for roasting
1 tsp ground coriander
salt and pepper

For the dressing
½ red chilli, finely chopped
½ garlic clove, crushed
½ small bunch of coriander, finely chopped

Preheat the oven to 200°C/gas mark 6.

Slice the narrow end of the butternut squash into slices around 5mm thick (no need to peel). Halve each slice, so you have half-moon shapes. Place in a roasting tin, drizzle with olive oil, sprinkle with the ground coriander and season well with salt and pepper. Roast in the oven for 25 minutes.

Meanwhile, make the dressing by whisking the chilli, garlic, 1 tbsp olive oil and chopped coriander together with a fork. Spoon this over the squash and serve hot or cold.

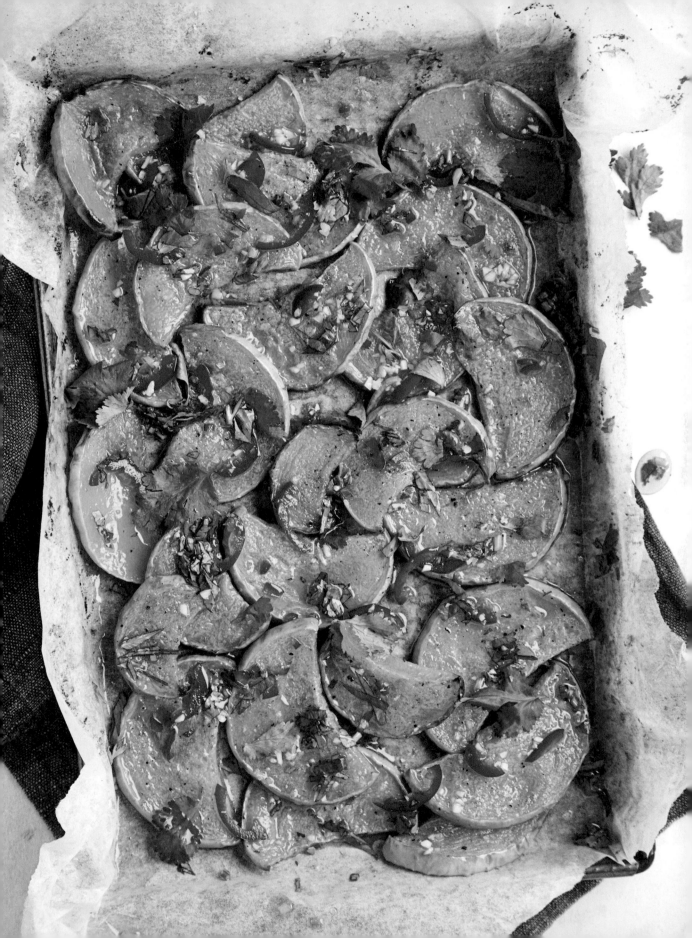

FAT (G): 12.4
PROTEIN (G): 5.2
SUGAR (G): 9.3
FIBRE (G): 3.6
KCAL: 179
SERVES: 2

This fresh, crunchy salad goes with just about anything. As with the Garlicky Green Veg (see page 68), the sweet and zesty dressing here would be delicious served with any green vegetables, hot or cold.

BROCCOLI & COURGETTE SALAD WITH PEANUT DRESSING

125g Tenderstem broccoli
1 small courgette, shaved into ribbons
    using a potato peeler
1 tbsp toasted sesame seeds, to serve

For the dressing
2 tsp peanut butter
1 tbsp olive oil
2 tsp cider vinegar
juice of ½ lemon
2 tsp honey

"Refreshing steamed green vegetables in cold water helps them retain their vibrant colour and a nice crunch – particularly good if using in a salad. After draining them, plunge them straight into cold water."

Steam the Tenderstem broccoli over simmering water for 5 minutes, then refresh by placing under running cold water. Drain again. Arrange the ribbons of courgette and cooked broccoli on a serving dish.

Make the dressing by whisking together all the ingredients. To serve, drizzle the dressing over the vegetables and top with the sesame seeds.

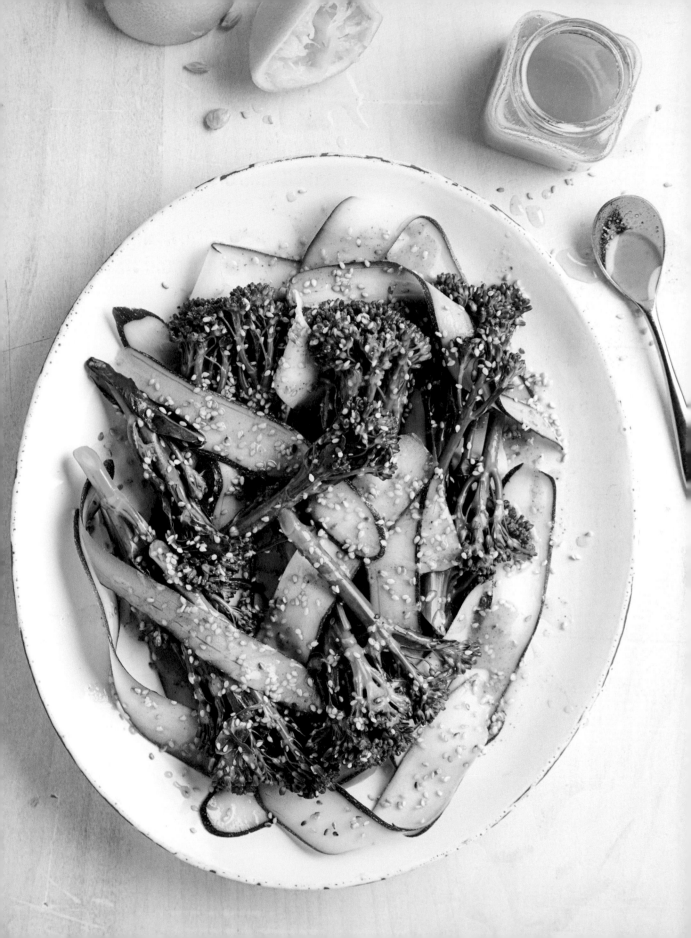

FAT (G): 7
PROTEIN (G): 2.6
SUGAR (G): 8
FIBRE (G): 3.9
KCAL: 121
SERVES: 2

Georgie is a coleslaw snob, which I admire, although I'll even eat school lunch coleslaw quite happily. This recipe is the best though: simple, Asian flavours. It packs a big hit of nutrients with the trio of raw vegetables and wonderfully tangy dressing. Perfect served with a piece of fish or meat. This also keeps well in the fridge for a day or so, unlike a lot of salads.

ASIAN RED CABBAGE, CARROT & SPINACH SLAW

200g red cabbage (about ½ small cabbage),
    finely sliced
1 small carrot, grated
50g spinach, roughly chopped
1 tbsp sesame oil
juice of 1 lime
2 tsp soy sauce
1 tsp honey

Combine the cabbage, carrot and spinach together in a serving bowl.

In a separate bowl or mug, whisk the sesame oil, lime juice, soy sauce and honey together with a fork.

Pour the dressing over the salad and mix well before serving.

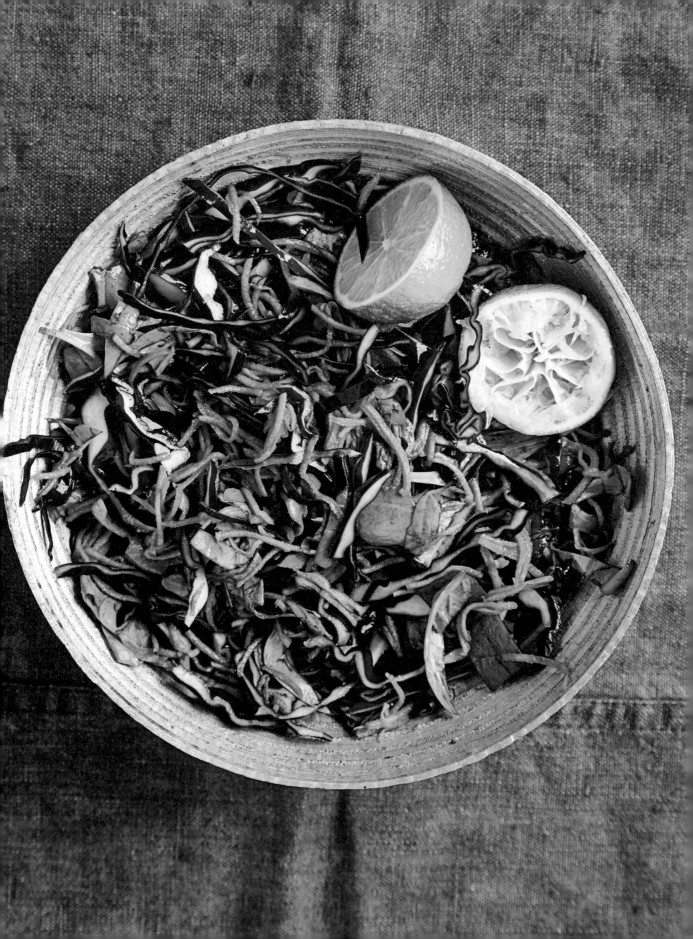

FAT (G): 20.1
PROTEIN (G): 4.9
SUGAR (G): 2.1
FIBRE (G): 11.8
KCAL: 259
SERVES: 2

A lovely, crunchy salad that goes well with almost anything. Stir through some cooked quinoa and you have yourself a complete meal.

AVOCADO, FENNEL & ASPARAGUS SALAD

125g fine asparagus spears
1 avocado
1 fennel bulb
juice of 1 lemon
Dijon Dressing (see page 57), to serve

"To roast the asparagus instead of steaming, I just toss the spears in oil and salt and stick them in the oven preheated to a high temperature. Then I forget about them. You'll eventually smell burning and then they'll be crunchy and amazing."

Steam the asparagus over simmering water for 3–4 minutes until just tender, then refresh by placing under lots of running cold water.

Peel, stone and slice the avocado, and slice the fennel, then immediately toss both in the lemon juice to prevent them turning brown. Top with the asparagus spears and serve with the Dijon Dressing.

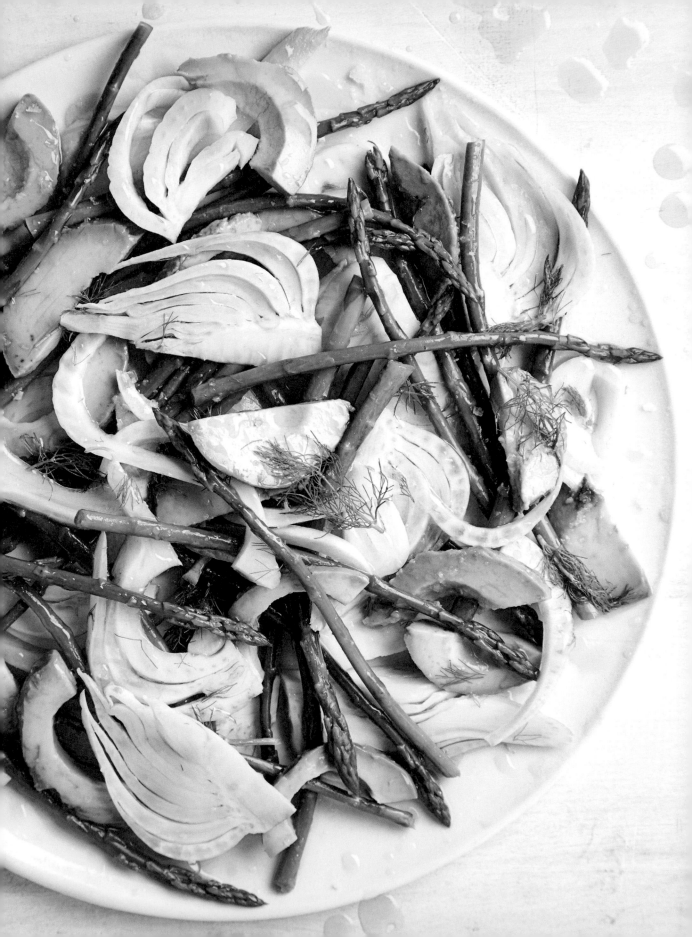

FAT (G): 14.3
PROTEIN (G): 1.9
SUGAR (G): 0.7
FIBRE (G): 1
KCAL: 147
SERVES: 2

This is a really simple but great combination of steamed and raw greens. Use any salad leaves (I like bitter leaves such as rocket, frisée, watercress and radicchio), and swap kale for spinach, Tenderstem broccoli or green beans, if you prefer.

STEAMED VEGETABLES & BITTER GREENS

75g kale, coarse stalks removed
50g rocket leaves
Simple Lemon Dressing (see page 57)

"If you've pan-fried anything to go with this – fish, steak, pork chops, eggs and so on – then just throw the steamed greens into the hot fat for a minute or so. It'll both make the pan easier to clean and make the veg taste great."

Steam the kale over simmering water for 2 minutes until just wilted. Tip on top of the rocket leaves (so the rocket wilts slightly) and dress with the Simple Lemon Dressing. Serve immediately.

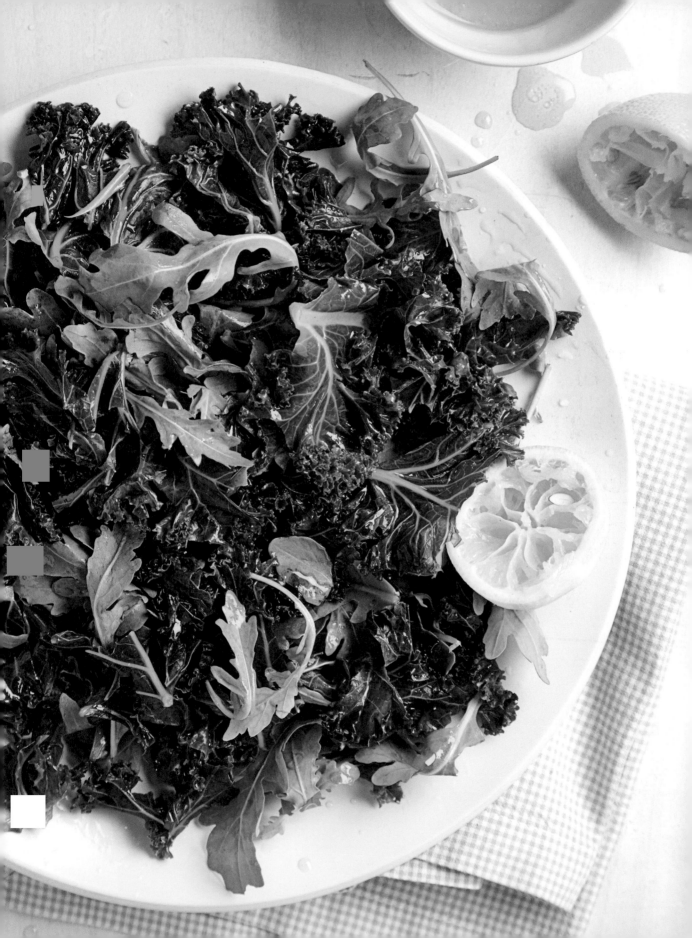

FAT (G): 7.3
PROTEIN (G): 2.1
SUGAR (G): 1.9
FIBRE (G): 3.5
KCAL: 99
SERVES: 2

You could really use any green vegetable here. Georgie likes beans. The combination of olive oil, garlic and lemon juice transforms the beans from mundane to magnificent and will certainly make it easier (and yummier) to load your plate up with vegetables.

GARLICKY GREEN VEG

200g green beans
1 tbsp olive oil
1 or more garlic cloves, chopped or smashed,
    to taste
juice of 1 lemon
salt and pepper

Steam the green beans over simmering water for 5 minutes, or until just cooked. They should still be crunchy. (Or just throw them into the hot oil with the garlic if you're lazy.)

Heat the olive oil in a pan over a low heat, add the garlic and cook for 1 minute, then add the lemon juice, cooked beans (if you steamed them first), salt and pepper. Quickly toss everything in the pan and serve.

FAT (G): 9.2
PROTEIN (G): 17.3
SUGAR (G): 4
FIBRE (G): 12.3
KCAL: 347
SERVES: 2

A super-quick storecupboard side and a wonderful alternative to mashed potato. Serve this topped with Spiced Roast Roots (see page 82), a handful of rocket and a good drizzle of olive oil for a delicious and comforting supper.

WHITE BEAN MASH

1 tbsp olive oil
1 garlic clove, chopped
2 x 400g cans of cannellini or butter beans
    (drained weight 500g), rinsed
100ml water
salt and pepper
juice of ½ lemon

Heat the oil in a pan over a low heat and fry the garlic for 2 minutes. Add the beans and water to the pan, increase the heat and cook for a further 2 minutes. Season well with salt, pepper and the lemon juice. Mash with a potato masher, or pulse in a food processor for a smoother mash.

FAT (G): 7.6
PROTEIN (G): 5
SUGAR (G): 5.6
FIBRE (G): 4.1
KCAL: 148
SERVES: 2

An interesting, nutritionally dense and pretty salad. Serve with simply steamed salmon or poached eggs.

ROAST RADISH, BROCCOLI & KALE SALAD

85g radishes, halved
½ head of broccoli (about 200g), roughly chopped
salt and pepper
1 tbsp olive oil, plus more for roasting
75g kale, coarse stalks removed
1 tbsp natural yogurt
juice of 1 lemon
50g pomegranate seeds

Preheat the oven to 180°C/gas mark 4.

Place the radishes and broccoli into a baking tray, season well with salt and pepper and drizzle with a little olive oil. Roast in the oven for 20 minutes. Add the kale to the baking tray and mix well. Return to the oven for a further 5 minutes.

Meanwhile, whisk the yogurt, 1 tbsp olive oil and lemon juice together to make a dressing. Transfer the roasted radishes, broccoli and kale to a serving dish, sprinkle over the pomegranate seeds and drizzle with the dressing. Serve hot or cold.

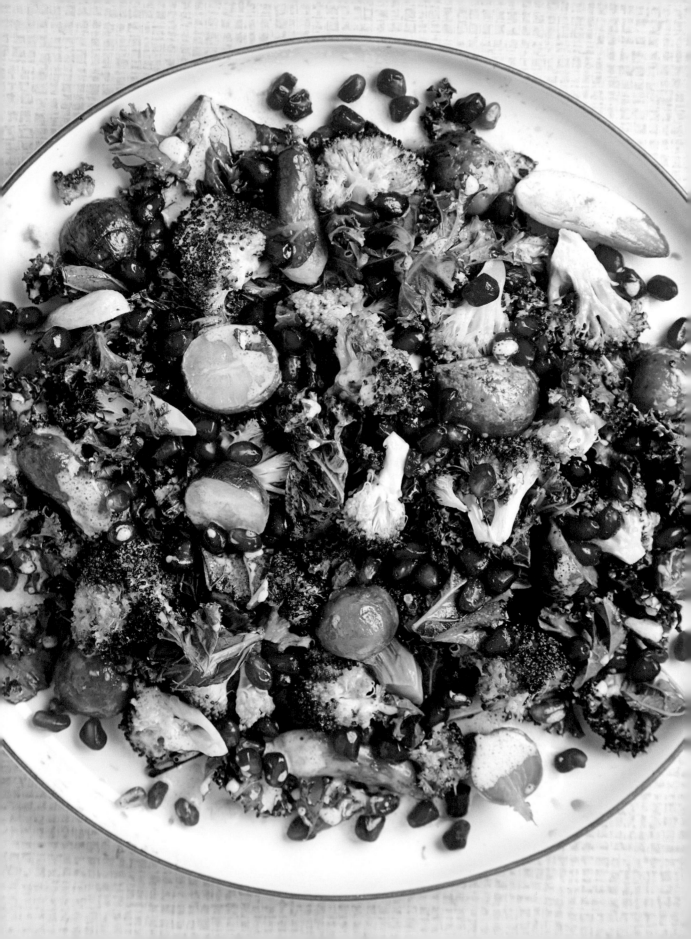

FAT (G): 22.4
PROTEIN (G): 9.2
SUGAR (G): 9.4
FIBRE (G): 7.7
KCAL: 290
SERVES: 2

The unusual bitter crunch of the chicory pairs well with the sweet orange and creamy walnuts in this dish. It's also a really eye-catching combination, great to serve to guests.

CHICORY, ORANGE & WALNUT SALAD

2 heads of red or green chicory, sliced into wedges
1 large orange, peeled and sliced
10g dill, coarse stalks removed, finely chopped
1 tbsp olive oil
juice of ½ lemon
50g walnuts, roughly chopped

Arrange the chicory and orange pieces on a serving dish.

In a small bowl, whisk together the dill, olive oil and lemon juice. Scatter the chopped walnuts over the salad and drizzle with the dressing just before serving.

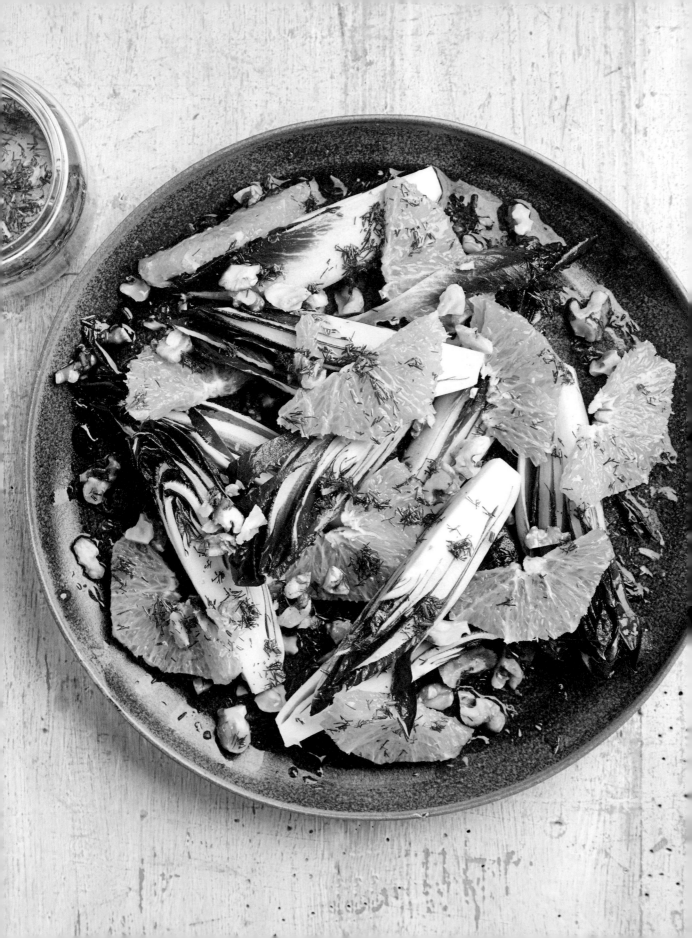

FAT (G): 5.6
PROTEIN (G): 6.1
SUGAR (G): 7.4
FIBRE (G): 6.3
KCAL: 144
SERVES: 2

A wonderful side dish that goes particularly well with roast chicken or lamb. Alternatively, serve as a light dinner, topped with two poached eggs. Braising the Little Gem is an exciting way to prepare the lettuces (particularly if they're looking a bit wilted at the back of the fridge): they retain a little crunch but take on a sweet, nutty flavour.

BRAISED LITTLE GEM & PEAS

drizzle of olive oil
1 bunch of spring onions, sliced
1 garlic clove, sliced
2 Little Gem lettuces, quartered
100ml vegetable or chicken stock
150g petits pois
salt and pepper
juice of 1 lemon

Heat the oil in a frying pan and sauté the spring onions for 5 minutes, until soft and translucent. Add the garlic and cook for another minute before adding the Little Gems and stock. Simmer for 5 minutes, until the lettuces are beginning to soften.

Add the peas, cover with a lid and cook for a further couple of minutes until the peas are just cooked. Season well with salt and pepper, squeeze over the lemon juice and serve.

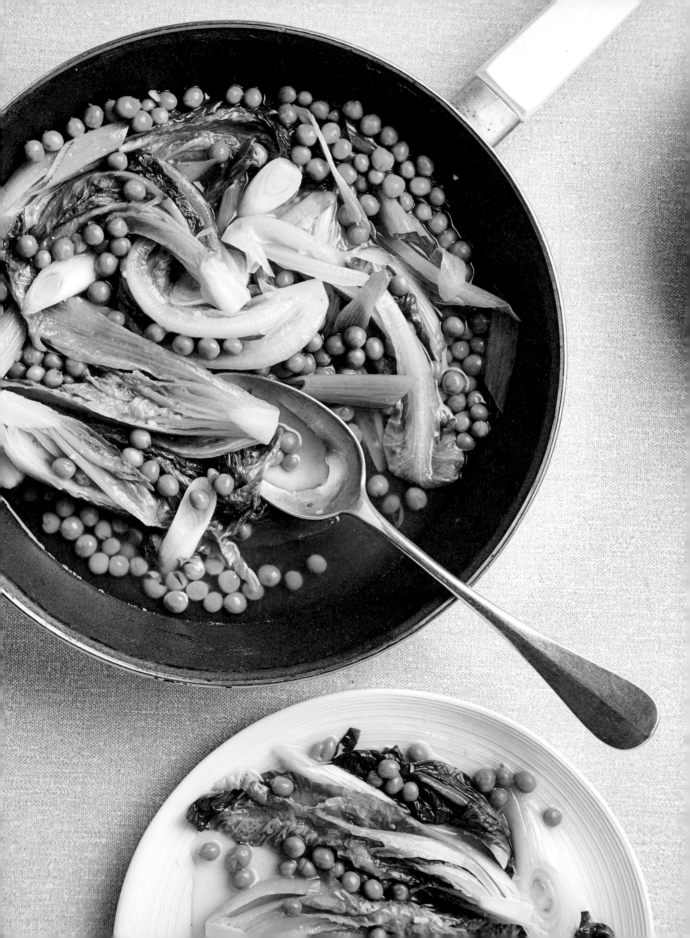

FAT (G): 8
PROTEIN (G): 6.4
SUGAR (G): 4.4
FIBRE (G): 5.4
KCAL: 140
SERVES: 2

Another great potato alternative and
a fun way to serve broccoli.

BROCCOLI & BASIL MASH

1 head of broccoli, roughly
    chopped (including the stalk)
10g basil
1 heaped tbsp natural yogurt
juice of 1 lemon
1 tbsp olive oil
salt and pepper

Steam the broccoli over simmering water for
10 minutes until soft. Place the broccoli and
remaining ingredients into a food processor
and pulse-blend until combined.

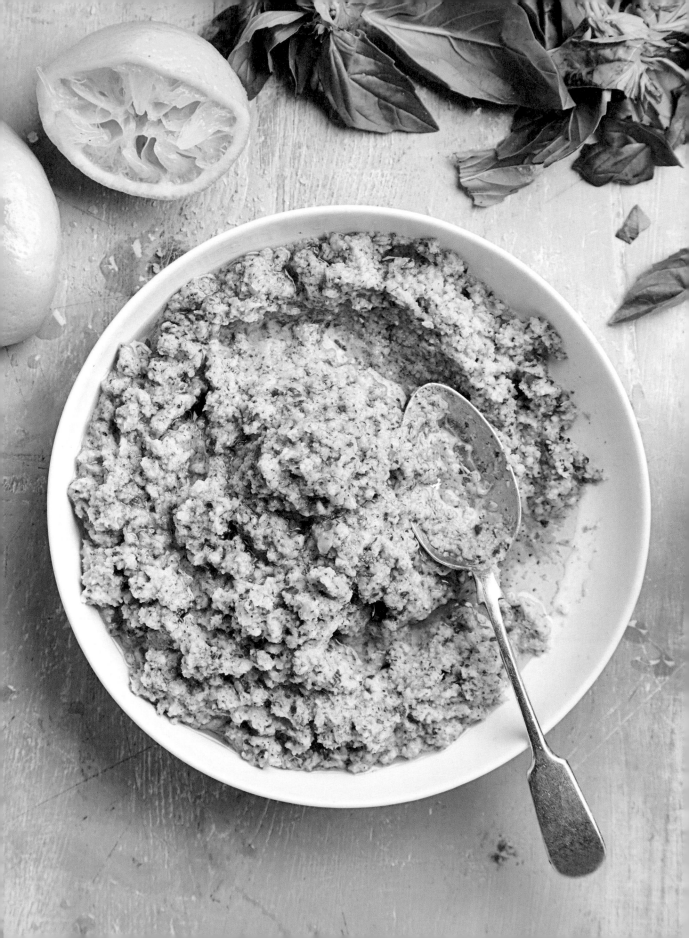

FAT (G): 10.5
PROTEIN (G): 5.4
SUGAR (G): 18.3
FIBRE (G): 10.4
KCAL: 225
SERVES: 2

Miso is a Japanese paste made from fermented soy beans. It is rich and deeply savoury and adds an amazing depth to dishes. This roast aubergine is one of my favourite vegetable dishes and a real crowd-pleaser.

MISO AUBERGINE

1 aubergine
2 tbsp miso paste (whichever type you can find)
juice of 1 lime
1 tbsp honey
1 tbsp sesame oil
1 tbsp sesame seeds (optional)
1 tbsp pomegranate seeds (optional)

Preheat the oven to 160°C/gas mark 3 and line a roasting tray with foil or baking parchment (this is because the miso mixture is a pain to scrub off).

Cut the aubergine in half, then split each half lengthways, then cut each piece into wedges. Score each piece roughly with a knife. Combine the miso paste, lime juice, honey and sesame oil in a small bowl.

Put the aubergine in the lined roasting tray and pour over the miso dressing, mixing well so each piece is covered. Roast in the oven for 40 minutes until soft.

Sprinkle with the sesame and pomegranate seeds, if using, and serve.

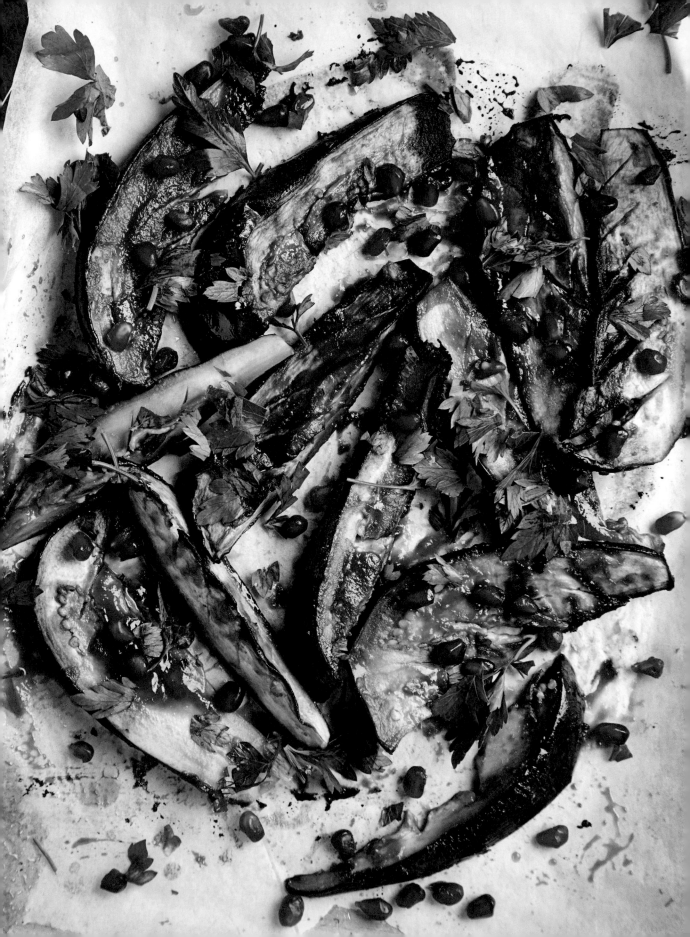

FAT (G): 11.5
PROTEIN (G): 8.8
SUGAR (G): 4.8
FIBRE (G): 10
KCAL: 247
SERVES: 2

Quinoa is a great grain substitute and a versatile plant-protein source for vegetarians. This recipe is a wonderful side dish for any meat or fish, in place of white carbohydrates.

"Although quinoa is used and cooked like a grain, it is actually a seed packed with lots of plant-protein."

QUINOA TABBOULEH

50g quinoa
500ml stock
1 courgette, finely chopped
2 tomatoes (about 125g), finely chopped
finely grated zest and juice of 1 unwaxed lemon
30g herb leaves (I like a mixture of flat-leaf parsley, mint and coriander), chopped
1 tsp tahini
1 tbsp olive oil
salt and pepper

Put the quinoa in a small saucepan with the stock. Bring to the boil, then reduce the heat to a simmer and cook for 15–20 minutes. Drain and rinse well with lots of cold water.

Place the quinoa into a serving bowl with the rest of the ingredients and mix everything together well, seasoning with salt and pepper.

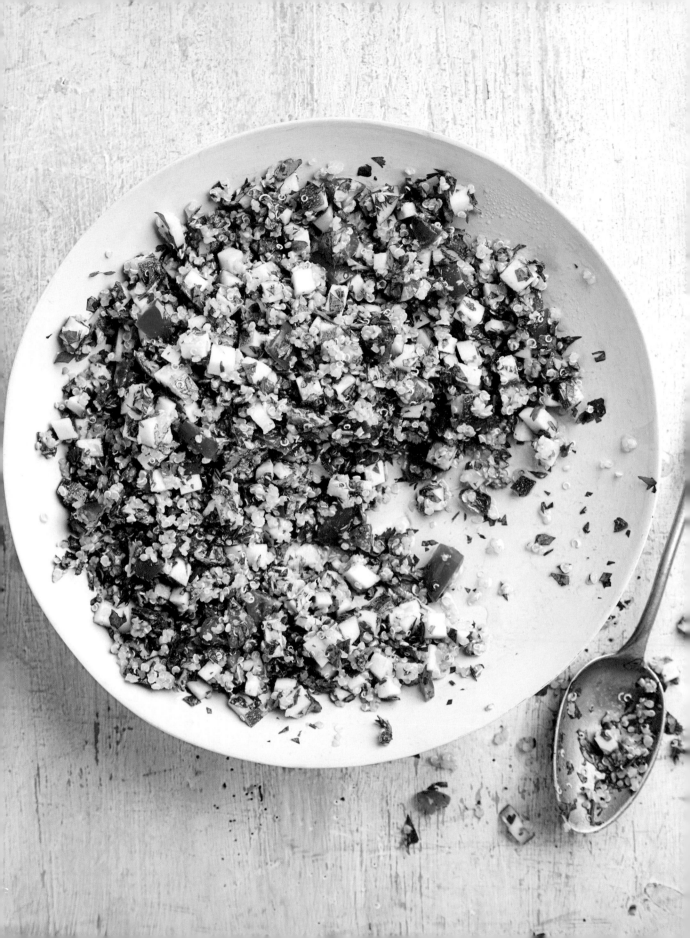

FAT (G): 7.8
PROTEIN (G): 4.2
SUGAR (G): 17.4
FIBRE (G): 9
KCAL: 214
SERVES: 2

I love the smoky spice of these roasted vegetables. Serve with any meat or fish, or top with two poached eggs, add some salad leaves and you have yourself a delicious dinner.

SPICED ROAST ROOTS

2 tbsp tomato purée
pinch of chilli flakes
1 tbsp olive oil
1 tsp paprika
1 tsp ground coriander
juice of 1 lemon
salt and pepper
1 beetroot, peeled and cut into small wedges
2 carrots, sliced into diagonal wedges
1 parsnip, sliced into diagonal wedges
leaves from a small bunch of flat-leaf parsley, chopped (optional)

Preheat the oven to 180°C/gas mark 4.

In a small bowl, combine the tomato purée, chilli flakes, olive oil, paprika, ground coriander and lemon juice. Season well with salt and pepper.

Put the vegetables and spice mix into a roasting tray, mixing well to ensure that all the vegetables are coated. Roast in the oven for 40–45 minutes, until soft but with a little bite. Sprinkle with parsley, if you like.

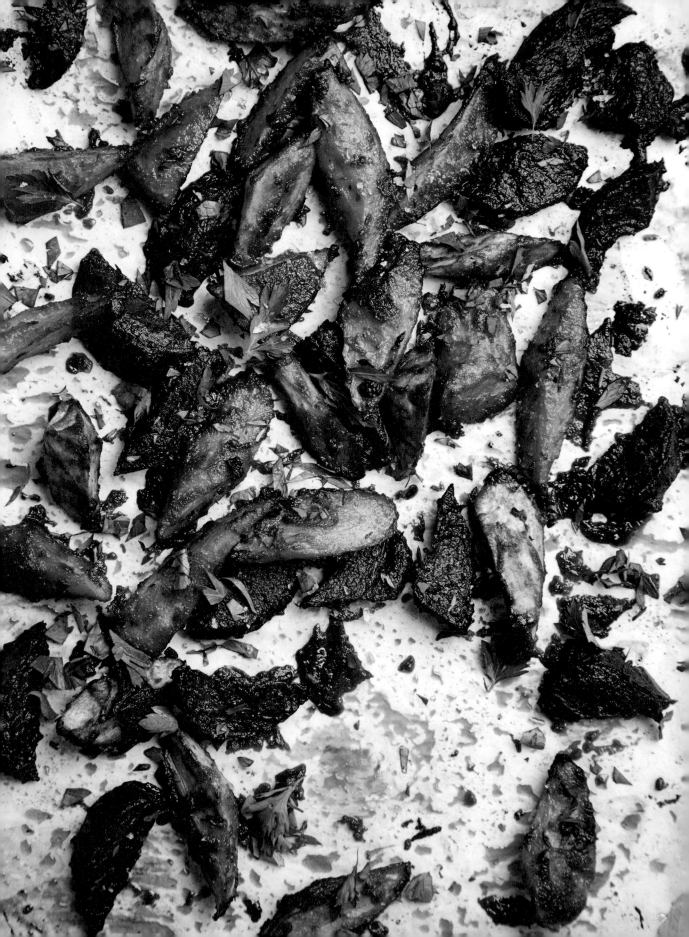

FAT (G): 10.7
PROTEIN (G): 4.6
SUGAR (G): 23.7
FIBRE (G): 10.3
KCAL: 254
SERVES: 2

Slow-cooked, lightly spiced red cabbage is a wonderful winter's dish. It also keeps, reheats and freezes really well (unlike most vegetables). Pair with Slow-Roast Shoulder of Pork (see page 106).

BRAISED RED CABBAGE

½ large red cabbage (around 400g), sliced
1 small fennel bulb, sliced
150ml water
1 tbsp white wine vinegar
1 heaped tsp ground cinnamon
25g unsalted butter
1 tbsp honey
salt and pepper

Preheat the oven to 160°C/gas mark 3.

Place all the ingredients in a small ovenproof dish, cover with foil and cook in the oven for 2 hours (stirring a couple of times during cooking), until the vegetables are soft and infused with the flavours.

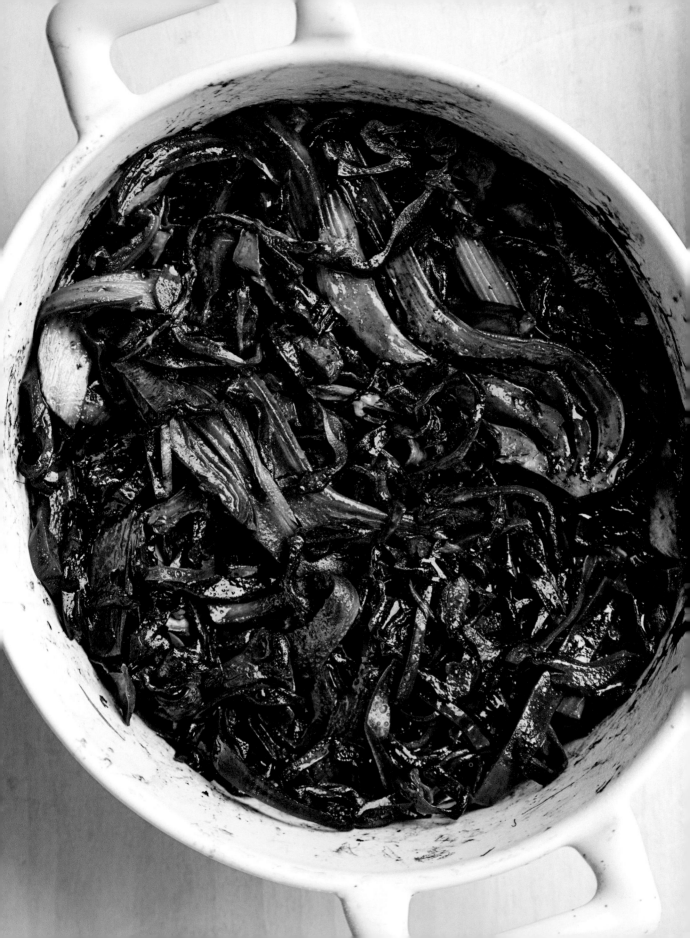

FAT (G): 12.7
PROTEIN (G): 19.7
SUGAR (G): 22.1
FIBRE (G): 27.6
KCAL: 450
SERVES: 2

This makes an excellent one-tray light lunch or supper for two, great with a big dollop of Greek yogurt. For something a little more filling, stir through brown rice or quinoa, or serve with a baked salmon fillet on top.

SPICED CHICKPEA & AUBERGINE RATATOUILLE

1 aubergine, cubed
400g can of tomatoes
1 tsp ground cumin
1 tsp ground cinnamon
3 garlic cloves, chopped
1 tbsp sunflower oil
salt and pepper
120g drained, canned chickpeas, rinsed
    (i.e. a 400g can)
chopped coriander, parsley or basil leaves, to serve
finely grated zest and juice of 1 unwaxed lemon
1 courgette, grated

Preheat the oven to 180°C/gas mark 4.

Place the aubergine, tomatoes, ground cumin and cinnamon, garlic and sunflower oil into a baking tray and mix well. Season well with salt and pepper. Roast in the oven for 35 minutes.

Add the drained chickpeas, stir well and return to the oven for another 10 minutes.

Remove from the oven and stir through the herbs, lemon zest and juice and courgette.

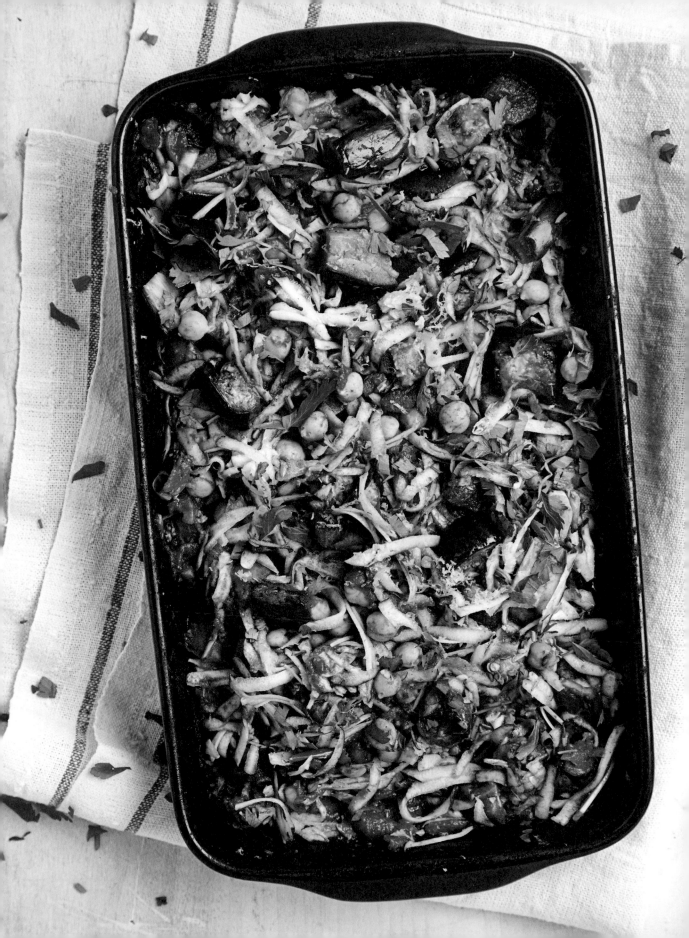

FAT (G): 7.2
PROTEIN (G): 2.4
SUGAR (G): 7.3
FIBRE (G): 3.8
KCAL: 166
SERVES: 2

Swap frozen chips for these sweet potato versions. This is a great technique for getting your chips nice and crispy. Keep the skins on for added fibre.

CRISPY SWEET POTATO CHIPS

1 large sweet potato (or 2 small), washed and
   cut into thin wedges
pinch of salt
1 heaped tsp cornflour
1 tbsp olive oil

Place the sweet potato in a large bowl of cold water for 1 hour (or more); this draws out some of the starch leading to a crispier chip. When ready to cook, preheat the oven to 200°C/gas mark 6.

Drain the chips well and pat dry with kitchen paper. Place the chips in a large bowl with the rest of the ingredients and mix well with your hands so that each piece of potato is coated. Lay on a baking tray (making sure you don't overcrowd the tray; use 2 if you need to), then cook in the oven for 15 minutes.

Now turn the chips with a spatula and cook for a further 15–20 minutes.

DIPS

Make up a batch of your favourite dip at the weekend and enjoy during the week with raw vegetables, or thickly spread on toast. Or serve any of them alongside simple vegetables, meat or fish to liven up your dinner.

AVOCADO HOUMOUS

1 avocado, peeled and stoned
120g drained, canned chickpeas, rinsed
    (i.e. a 400g can)
2 tsp tahini
juice of 1 lemon
1 tbsp olive oil
½ garlic clove
salt and pepper

Put all the ingredients into a food processor and pulse until smooth.

BEETROOT, CASHEW & SESAME

75g cashew nuts, soaked in warm
    water for at least 30 minutes
150g beetroot (raw or cooked)
50g natural yogurt
1 tsp sesame oil
juice of ½ lemon
salt and pepper

Drain the nuts and place in a food processor with the rest of the ingredients. Blend until smooth.

TZATZIKI

125g cucumber, grated and squeezed in a clean
    tea towel to get rid of the excess water
1 small garlic clove, chopped
150g natural yogurt
salt and pepper

Combine all the ingredients together well in a small bowl.

OLIVE TAPENADE

200g black olives, pitted
1 garlic clove
juice of 1 lemon
2 tbsp capers
small bunch of flat-leaf parsley
salt and pepper
3 tbsp olive oil, plus more if needed

Place all the ingredients into a food processor and process until smooth, adding a little more olive oil if necessary.

MEAT

Meat is our most maligned food group – particularly red meat. It's held responsible for heart disease, cancer and climate change. You should really only worry about one of these (climate change). You're made of meat and so you can live off it. That doesn't mean you should, but it's worth noting that a decent steak has everything you need – in other words, it's nutritionally complete. I spent some time in the Arctic and Russia, where people did live off red meat (mostly whale, deer and walrus if you're curious). There are very few vegetables that grow inside the Arctic Circle and so their diet was exceptionally high in fat and high in protein. Stories abound about how healthy this diet is and certainly the residents of the region lived longer than you might expect, though the effects of long winters, smoking, alcohol and violence took their toll. The only meat you couldn't live off is rabbit. Rabbits, for reasons best known to themselves and a few rabbit experts (cuniculturists, if you must know) have extremely lean meat. As many early Polar explorers found to their cost, man cannot live off rabbit alone. You need fat to live.

HOW TO COOK THE PERFECT STEAK

Remembering a couple of key tips is crucial to cooking a steak well. I favour a sirloin steak, as it's really flavoursome but still tender. Go for fillet for a special occasion, or rump for a cheaper option. Adjust the cooking time depending on the thickness of your steak, but always remember the following:

Ensure your steak is at room temperature
Dry your meat well
Oil and season the meat, not the pan
Allow the meat to rest for 3–5 minutes
Don't cook more than 2 steaks in a pan

1 sirloin steak (about 2cm thick)
1 tbsp olive oil
salt and pepper

Remove the steak from the fridge and allow it to come up to room temperature before you cook it (this takes 20–30 minutes).

Dry your steak well with kitchen paper (this helps create a lovely golden crust), rub it with the olive oil on both sides and season with salt and pepper.

Heat a frying pan over a high heat and ensure it is really hot; you want to hear that sizzle as the meat hits the pan. Place your steak in the pan and cook for 1–5 minutes each side depending on how you like it (see below). Only turn the steaks once during the cooking; you want each side to have time to really caramelize.

Remove the steak from the pan and place on a board to rest for 3–5 minutes. Resting the meat allows the juices to absorb back into the meat, resulting in a juicy, flavoursome steak.

Approximate cooking times for a 2cm thick steak:

Blue: About 1 minute each side
Rare: About 1½ minutes each side
Medium-rare: About 2 minutes each side
Medium: About 2¼ minutes each side
Well-done: 4–5 minutes each side

You can check your steak by making a small incision with a knife (remember it will continue to cook slightly as it rests). I prefer to check by prodding it with my finger: the meat feels really soft when rare; medium-rare it firms up slightly and becomes a little bouncier; well-done will be much firmer. You will soon remember how your ideal steak feels to the touch, making it quick and easy to judge when it's done.

SAUCES

These sauces are so delicious. Perfect with meat, but also great with fish and vegetables. Put all the ingredients in a food processor and whizz until smooth. They keep in the fridge for up to 1 week.

SALSA VERDE

½ garlic clove
1 tsp Dijon mustard
1 tbsp capers (about 15g)
juice of 1 lemon
50g herbs (I like to
    use flat-leaf parsley,
    coriander and basil)
4 tbsp olive oil

ROMESCO

75g jarred roast
    red peppers,
    drained weight
½ garlic clove
35g almonds
juice of 1 lemon
2 tbsp olive oil
pinch of salt and pepper

CHIMICHURRI

1 spring onion
½ garlic clove
20g coriander
20g flat-leaf parsley
1 red chilli, stalk removed
   and deseeded
4 tbsp olive oil
1 tbsp cider vinegar

FAT (G): 14.9
PROTEIN (G): 73.2
SUGAR (G): 1.6
FIBRE (G): 2.4
CALORIES: 463
SERVES: 4

A simple roast chicken is a wonderful thing. It's a cost-effective weekend family meal but equally lovely cooked for fewer people with lots of leftover meat to enjoy during the week.

SIMPLE LEMON & HERB ROAST CHICKEN

1.5kg whole chicken
1 lemon
1 onion, halved
small bunch of thyme, tarragon or sage
2 tbsp olive oil
salt and pepper

Remove the chicken from the fridge 30 minutes before cooking, to allow it to come up to room temperature. Preheat the oven to 190°C/gas mark 5.

Snip off any string holding the chicken together and place it in a large roasting tin. Roll the lemon on a work surface (to release the juices) and stab it all over with a sharp knife. Stuff the lemon, onion and herbs inside the cavity of the chicken. Rub the olive oil over the breasts and legs and season well with salt and pepper.

Roast in the oven for approximately 1 hour 20 minutes, basting with the juices a couple of times during cooking. Check the meat is cooked by piercing the thigh: if the juices run clear, it is cooked. If not, cook for a few minutes more before checking again.

Place the chicken on a board and cover loosely with foil. Leave to rest for 10–15 minutes before carving.

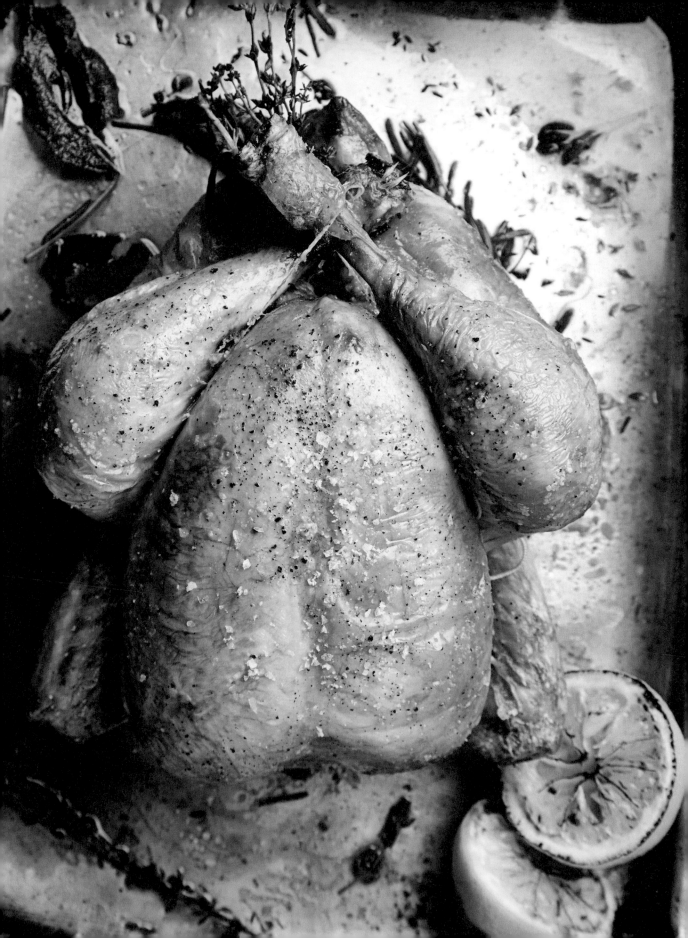

FAT (G): 14.9
PROTEIN (G): 73.3
SUGAR (G): 1.5
FIBRE (G): 1
CALORIES: 461
SERVES: 4

An easy but effective way of preparing a whole chicken. By removing the backbone you can flatten out the whole bird, meaning the marinade has a bigger surface area to permeate. It also reduces the cooking time.

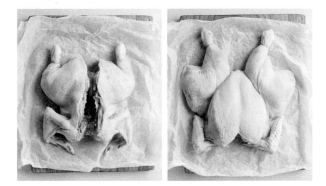

SPATCHCOCKED PAPRIKA SPICED ROAST CHICKEN

1.5kg whole chicken
6 garlic cloves, crushed
1 heaped tsp ground cumin
1 heaped tsp paprika
1 heaped tsp ground coriander
2 tbsp olive oil
finely grated zest and juice of 1 unwaxed lemon
1 red onion, roughly sliced
salt and pepper

Snip off any string holding the chicken together and place the bird, breast side down, on a chopping board with the legs facing away from you and wings facing towards you. Using a sharp pair of kitchen scissors, cut all the way down one side of the backbone and then all the way down the other side to remove the backbone. Turn the chicken over and press firmly down on the breast side to splay the bird out flat. Discard the backbone, or keep it for stock or gravy.

To make the marinade, mix together the garlic, cumin, paprika, coriander, olive oil and lemon zest and juice. Rub this all over the chicken (including underneath). Place the sliced onion in a large roasting tin, pop the chicken on top and season well with salt and pepper. Leave to marinate for 30 minutes, or overnight (the longer the better).

When ready to cook, preheat the oven to 190°C/gas mark 5 and roast the chicken for 45–50 minutes, or until the juices run clear and the meat is cooked. Baste with the juices 2–3 times during cooking.

Check the meat is cooked by piercing the thigh meat: if the juices run clear, it is cooked. If not, cook for a few minutes more before checking again.

Place the chicken on a board and cover loosely with foil. Leave to rest for 10–15 minutes before carving.

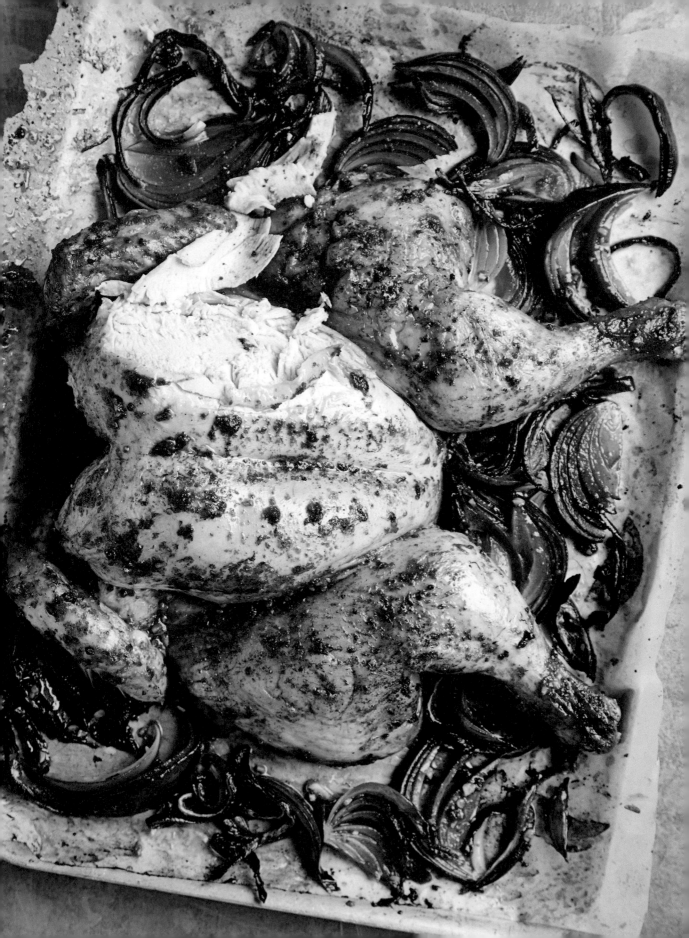

FAT (G): 17.8
PROTEIN (G): 36.5
SUGAR (G): 10.5
FIBRE (G): 7.6
CALORIES: 441
SERVES: 4

A lovely, rich beef recipe which goes wonderfully with White Bean Mash (see page 69) and a big pile of steamed greens. It keeps really well in the fridge for a few days and also freezes successfully.

SLOW-COOKED BEEF RAGÙ

1 tbsp olive oil
300g cubed stewing steak
1 onion, finely chopped
1 carrot, finely chopped
1 celery stick, finely chopped
3 garlic cloves, finely chopped
350g tomatoes, roughly chopped
1 glass of red wine (125ml)
200ml beef or lamb stock
2 tsp Worcestershire sauce
15g rosemary, leaves picked and roughly chopped
salt and pepper

Preheat the oven to 150°C/gas mark 2.

Heat the oil in a heavy-based pan over a medium-high heat and briefly sear the beef until just golden; do this in batches without overcrowding the pan. Remove the beef from the pan and set aside. Sauté the onion, carrot and celery in the same pan over a medium heat for 5–10 minutes until soft.

Next, add the garlic to the pan and sauté for another minute. Add the tomatoes and wine and cook for another 2–3 minutes until most of the liquid has evaporated. Put the beef back into the pan with the stock, Worcestershire sauce and rosemary. Season well with salt and pepper.

Place in the oven (without a lid) and leave to cook for 2 hours, checking regularly to ensure it's not drying out, adding a splash more water or stock if it is looking dry. After 2 hours, put the lid on and cook for a further 3 hours. The meat should now be really tender and falling apart. Remove from the oven and roughly shred the meat using 2 forks, then mix it back into the sauce and serve.

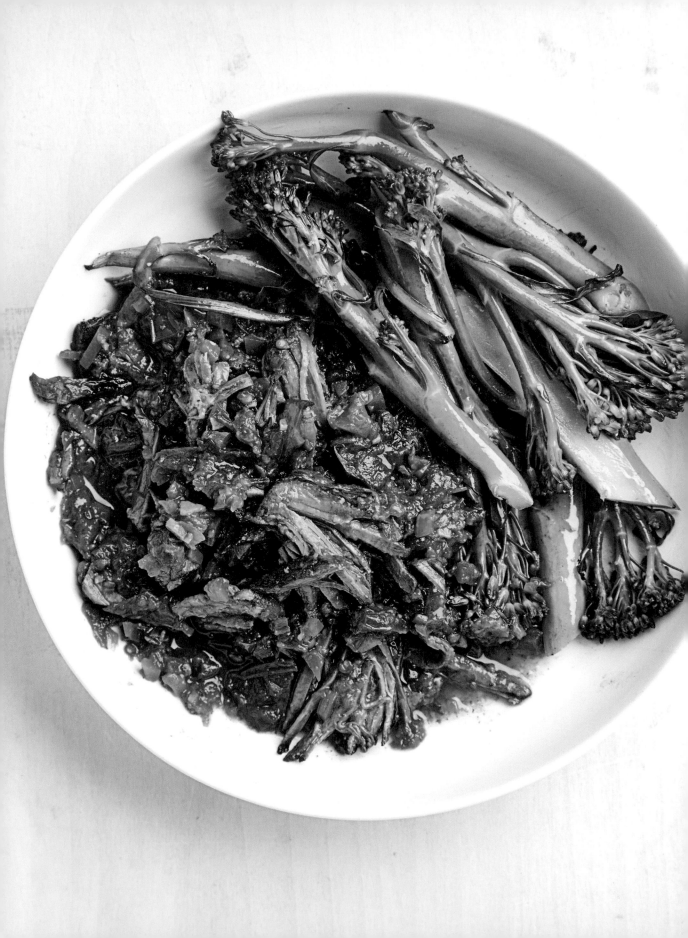

FAT (G): 22.3
PROTEIN (G): 60.1
SUGAR (G): 4
FIBRE (G): 1.7
CALORIES: 493
SERVES: 4

Chicken thighs are an excellent cut of meat, cheaper and more succulent than the breast. These are delicious served hot or cold.

TURMERIC TANDOORI CHICKEN THIGHS

2 tbsp natural yogurt
1 heaped tsp ground turmeric
1 heaped tsp garam masala, or curry powder
1 red chilli, sliced
4 garlic cloves, sliced
finely grated zest and juice of 1 unwaxed lemon
salt and pepper
1 red onion, sliced
drizzle of olive oil
4 chicken thighs

Make the marinade by mixing the yogurt, turmeric, garam masala, chilli, garlic, lemon zest and juice together in a bowl. Season well with salt and pepper.

Lay the sliced onion into an ovenproof dish, drizzle with olive oil and top with the chicken, stabbing the skin with a sharp knife to allow the marinade to permeate the meat. Pour the marinade over the chicken and onion and give it a good mix. Cover with cling film and leave to marinate in the fridge for at least 1 hour, preferably overnight.

When you're ready to cook, preheat the oven to 180°C/gas mark 4. Remove the chicken from the fridge and ensure that each piece is still well coated in the marinade. Bake for 30 minutes, turning and basting a couple of times as it cooks. Increase the oven temperature to 200°C/gas mark 6 for a final 15 minutes to crisp up the skin.

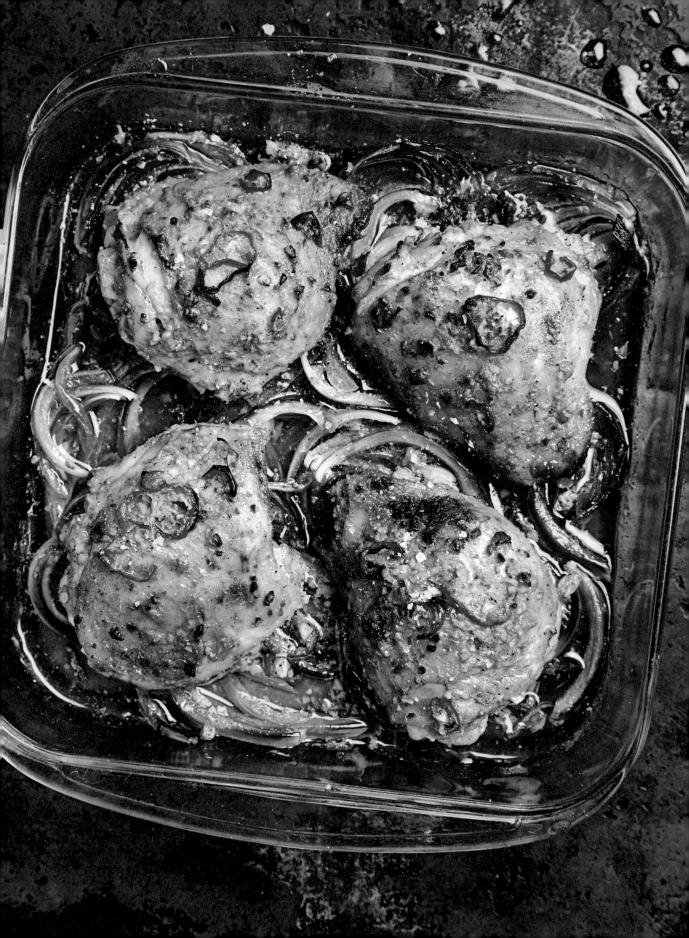

FAT (G): 15.1
PROTEIN (G): 5
SUGAR (G): 7.2
FIBRE (G): 6.2
CALORIES: 498
SERVES: 4

Pork and fennel is a wonderful combination. Cavolo nero is a really nutrient-dense vegetable and adds a lovely texture to the sauce.

PORK & FENNEL SEED MEATBALLS WITH CAVOLO NERO

For the meatballs
250g minced pork
3 spring onions, sliced
1 garlic clove, chopped
1 egg yolk
pinch of chilli flakes
1 heaped tsp fennel seeds, toasted in a dry pan
salt and pepper
1 tbsp olive oil
sliced chilli, to serve (optional)
finely grated Parmesan, to serve (optional)

For the sauce
2 garlic cloves, sliced
300g tomatoes, roughly chopped
150ml chicken or vegetable stock
150g cavolo nero or chard, stalks removed
   and roughly sliced
20g basil, leaves picked and roughly chopped
salt and pepper

Put all the ingredients for the meatballs (except the oil, chilli or Parmesan) into a large bowl, season with salt and pepper and mix well. Shape the mix into approximately 6–8 meatballs. Heat the oil in a pan and sear the meatballs for 1 minute each side until golden brown, then remove from the pan and set aside.

Using the same pan, sauté the garlic over a low heat for 1–2 minutes. Add the tomatoes, increase the heat and cook for 5 minutes until they start to break down, adding a splash of water if they are drying out. Add the stock and cavolo nero and simmer for 7–8 minutes. Season well with salt and pepper. Finally, add the meatballs, cover with a lid and simmer for another 5 minutes until they are cooked through. Sprinkle with basil and serve with chilli and Parmesan, if you like.

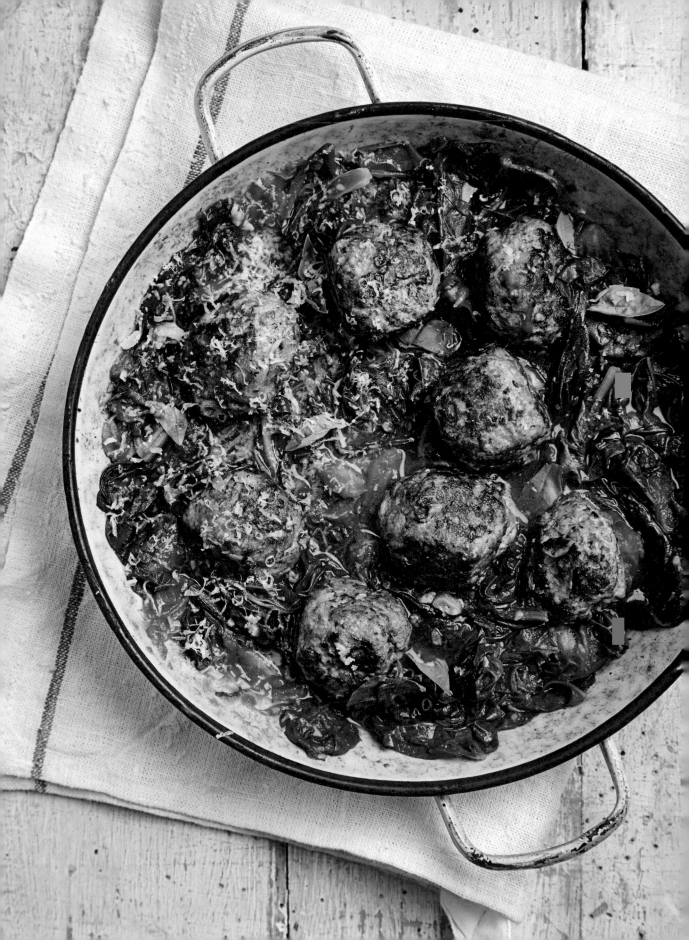

FAT (G): 8.9
PROTEIN (G): 53.7
SUGAR (G): 4.8
FIBRE (G): 4.1
CALORIES: 441
SERVES: 4

This is a simple but intensely comforting dish. The poached chicken is beautifully tender and the rice full of flavour from simmering in the stock. A great weekend dish to share with friends and family, or to cook and enjoy throughout the week ahead.

WHOLE POACHED CHICKEN

1 tbsp olive oil
1.5kg whole chicken
3 carrots, roughly chopped
2 leeks, roughly chopped
1 celery stick, roughly chopped
1.25 litres chicken stock
small bunch of flat-leaf parsley, thyme or dill
175g brown basmati rice
150g petits pois
100g spinach

Heat the olive oil in a large casserole dish. Snip off any string holding the chicken together, as well as any excess skin at either end of the bird. Place the chicken in the pan, breast side down, for 4–5 minutes to brown before flipping it back over. Drain off any excess oil and add the carrots and leeks to the pan with the celery, stock and herbs, reserving a few leaves to sprinkle over the finished dish. Clamp on a lid and bring to the boil, then reduce the heat to a slow simmer and cook for about 1 hour.

Check the chicken is cooked by puncturing the breast with a knife and ensuring the meat is no longer pink. If it is, cook for a few minutes more before checking again.

Remove the chicken from the pan and place on a plate, cover with foil and add the rice to the pan. Simmer for a further 25–30 minutes until the rice is cooked. A couple of minutes before the rice is ready, add the peas and spinach to the pan. Meanwhile, carve thick pieces of the poached chicken and put into bowls, spoon the rice, vegetables and stock over and serve.

FAT (G): 44.9
PROTEIN (G): 42.7
SUGAR (G): 3.6
FIBRE (G): 3.1
CALORIES: 812
SERVES: 4

The rules look strict: no junk food. But everyone has days when they want a blow-out. So we included this: our favourite, tastiest recipe regardless of calories, carbs or anything. Cook this rarely. It's amazing. It's still much better for you than a takeaway. Buy a nice Italian white to go with it.

SPAGHETTI CARBONARA

1 tbsp olive oil
8 rashers of pancetta or streaky bacon (about 125g), chopped
2 garlic cloves, sliced
salt and pepper
200g spaghetti
25g pecorino or Parmesan, finely grated
3 egg yolks

Heat the olive oil in a frying pan and fry the pancetta or bacon for 5–10 minutes until crisp. Reduce the heat, add the garlic and cook for another 2 minutes, then take off the heat and set aside.

Meanwhile, boil a large pan of salted water and cook the spaghetti according to the packet instructions.

In a small bowl, combine the pecorino or Parmesan with the egg yolks and season well with salt and lots of pepper.

Drain the spaghetti, reserving around ½ cup of the cooking water. Pour the cooked spaghetti into the pan with the bacon and heat very gently, stirring so it does not stick, adding the reserved cooking water to the pan to give a silky texture. Remove from the heat and mix through the egg yolks and cheese, then serve straight away.

FAT (G): 53.6
PROTEIN (G): 58.8
SUGAR (G): 7.9
FIBRE (G): 2.3
CALORIES: 776
SERVES: 4–6

An easy recipe that yields succulent, flavoursome meat with crisp crackling. A recipe to cook at the weekend and enjoy with friends. It goes excellently with the Braised Red Cabbage and Garlicky Green Veg (see pages 84 and 68).

SLOW-ROAST SHOULDER OF PORK

1.5kg pork shoulder (ask your butcher to score the skin)
sea salt flakes
2 red onions, sliced
2 apples, sliced

Preheat the oven to 220°C/gas mark 7. Fill and boil the kettle.

Place the pork into a colander, skin side up, and pour the freshly boiled water all over the skin (this helps create crisp crackling). Place the pork into a roasting tin and dry the skin well with kitchen paper. Sprinkle the skin liberally with sea salt and roast in the oven for 30 minutes.

Remove the pork from the oven and reduce the oven temperature to 160°C/gas mark 3. Place the onions and apples in the tray around and underneath the pork and cover tightly with foil. Put back in the oven for a further 5 hours.

For the final 30 minutes, increase the oven temperature to 200°C/gas mark 6 to crisp up the crackling.

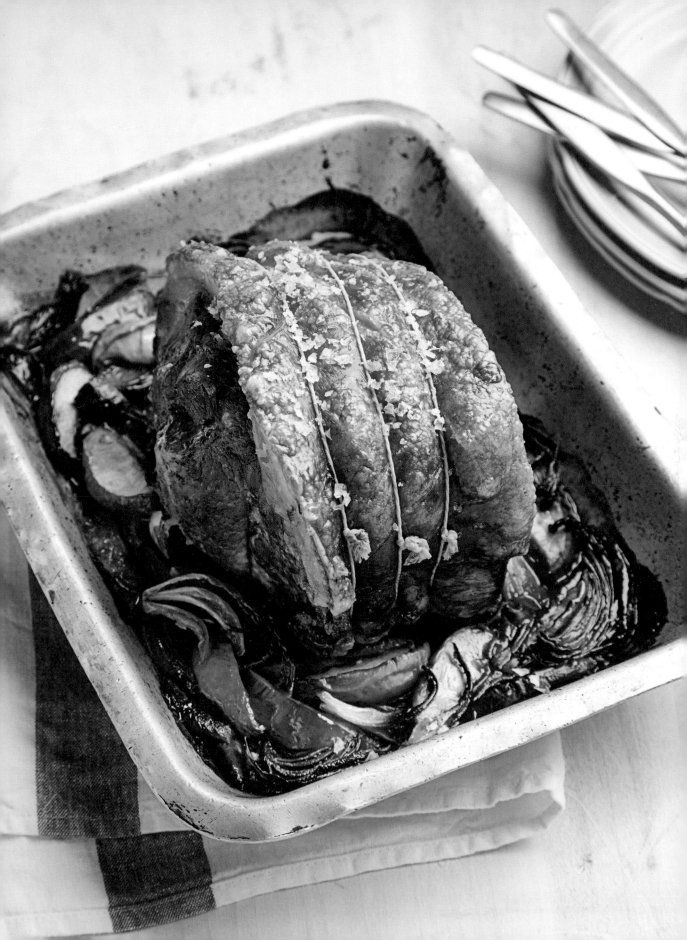

FAT (G): 26.7
PROTEIN (G): 53.5
SUGAR (G): 8.1
FIBRE (G): 2.7
CALORIES: 496
SERVES: 4

This is a simple but impressive dinner. (See page 91 for more on how to cook the perfect steak.)

ULTIMATE STEAK SALAD

2 Portobello mushrooms, sliced
250g cherry tomatoes, halved
1 tbsp olive oil
salt and pepper
1 large sirloin steak (around 300g) or 2 smaller ones, about 2cm thick
65g rocket, to serve

For the dressing
1 tbsp olive oil
1 tbsp balsamic vinegar
1 tsp horseradish sauce
drizzle of runny honey

> "I can't prove that it's healthier to eat fancy grass-fed steak, but I firmly believe it. I have spent time on both good and bad farms and it is impossible to believe that eating animals that are bulked up with steroids and antibiotics and spend their days miserable is going to be good for you."

Preheat the oven to 180°C/gas mark 4.

Put the mushrooms and tomatoes in a roasting tray, drizzle with 1 tbsp of olive oil and season well with salt and pepper. Roast for 25–30 minutes. Dry the steak well on both sides (this helps create a nice golden crust when frying), season well with salt and pepper on both sides and rub with a little olive oil.

Heat a frying pan over a high heat and fry the steak for 2 minutes each side (for medium-rare). Transfer to a board and leave it to rest for 5–10 minutes; this allows the meat to relax and become really tender.

For the dressing, whisk together the olive oil, balsamic vinegar, horseradish and honey and season well with salt and pepper.

To assemble the salad, arrange the rocket leaves, mushrooms and tomatoes on a serving plate and top with the slices of steak. Dress just before serving.

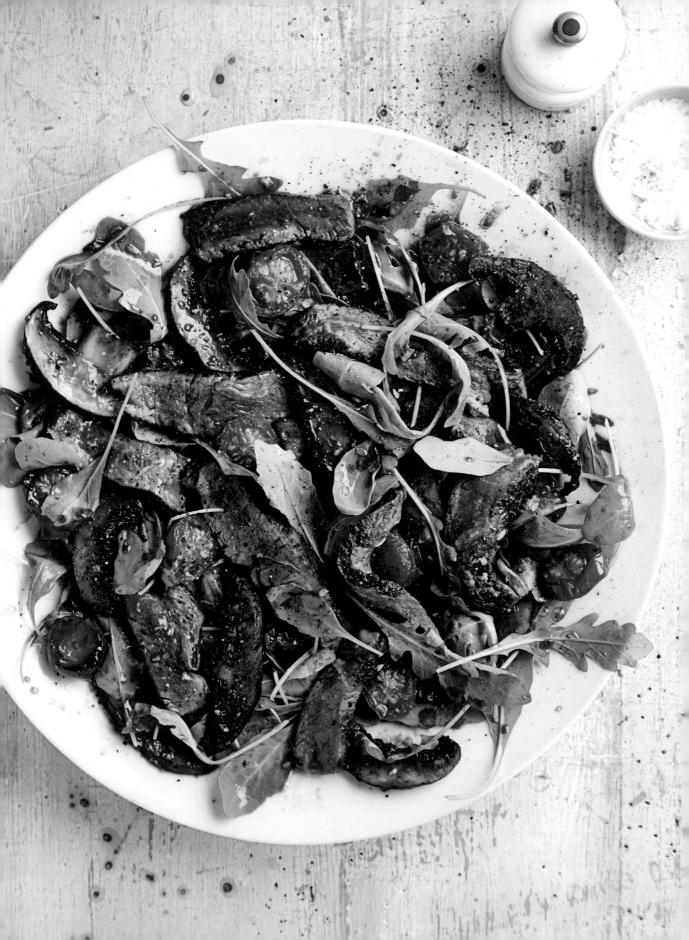

FAT (G): 24.1
PROTEIN (G): 71.8
SUGAR (G): 0.5
FIBRE (G): 1.5
CALORIES: 550
SERVES: 4

This is a simple and classic way to roast a leg of lamb. The garlic, rosemary and simple red wine gravy go perfectly with the sweet meat.

ROAST LEG OF LAMB WITH GARLIC & ROSEMARY

1 leg of lamb (about 1.5kg)
20g rosemary leaves, finely chopped
6 garlic cloves, finely chopped
4 anchovy fillets, finely chopped
2 tbsp olive oil
salt and pepper

For the gravy
1 tbsp plain flour
100ml red wine
750ml beef (or lamb) stock

Remove the leg of lamb from the fridge about 30 minutes before cooking to allow it to come to room temperature. Preheat the oven to 200°C/gas mark 6.

In a small bowl, mix together the rosemary, garlic, anchovies and olive oil and season well with salt and pepper. Place the lamb in a roasting tin and slice slits all over the top of it with a small knife (they should be just large enough to fit your fingertip into). Rub the garlic and rosemary mix all over the top of the lamb, working it into the incisions; this will penetrate the meat as it roasts and give it a wonderful flavour.

Cover the roasting tin with foil and place in the oven. Roast for 30 minutes, then remove the foil, reduce the oven temperature to 180°C/gas mark 4 and roast for a further 30 minutes (this will give you blushing pink meat; cook for a further 15–20 minutes if you like it well-done, but remember it will continue to cook slightly as it rests). Remove from the oven and place on a board to rest for 15–30 minutes.

To make the gravy, pour the juices from the roasting tin into a saucepan, add the flour and mix well over a medium heat. Add the wine and stir until thickened, then add the stock a little at a time, stirring as you go, until you have a smooth gravy. Serve with the lamb.

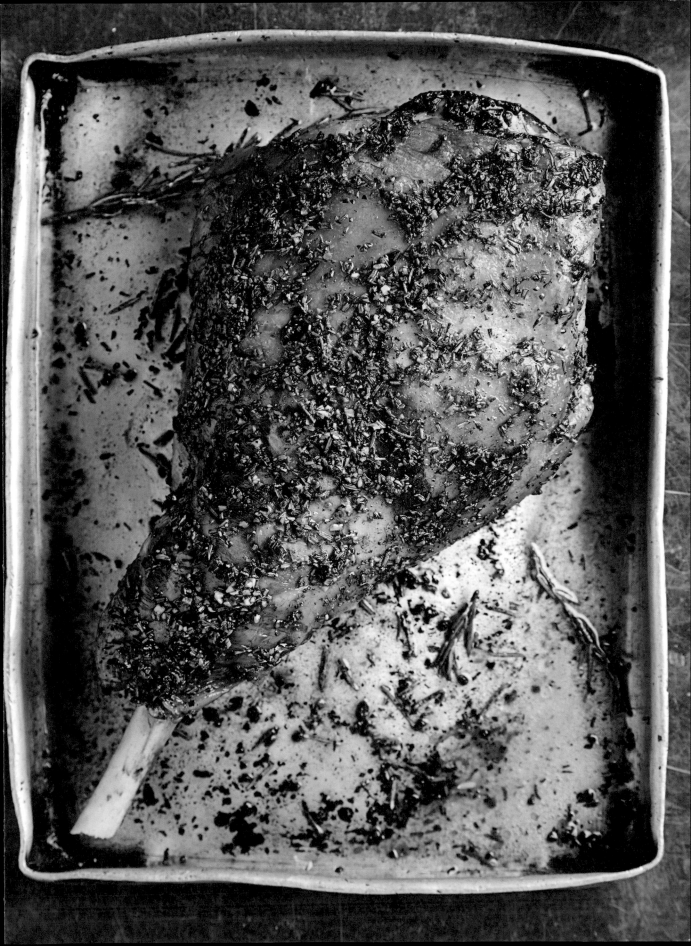

FAT (G): 31.4
PROTEIN (G): 56.9
SUGAR (G): 3
FIBRE (G): 7.9
CALORIES: 571
SERVES: 4

This makes a great midweek dinner, quick and easy to put together with ingredients you can grab on your way home from work. Kids love it, too, but leave the chilli out of theirs!

FIVE-SPICED BEEF IN LITTLE GEM WITH SMASHED AVOCADO

1 tbsp olive oil
350g minced beef
2 garlic cloves, chopped
3 tsp Chinese 5 spice
pinch of chilli flakes
1 avocado
juice of 1 lime
salt and pepper
2 Little Gem lettuces, separated into leaves
2 tbsp natural yogurt
small bunch of coriander, chopped

Heat the olive oil in a frying pan over a high heat, add the minced beef and cook, turning, until golden brown. Reduce the heat and add the garlic, 5 spice and chilli flakes, then mix well and cook for a further 2–3 minutes.

Meanwhile, peel and stone the avocado and mash with the lime juice in a small bowl, seasoning well with salt and pepper.

To serve, arrange the Little Gem leaves on a large plate, spoon the beef mixture into the lettuce leaves, then top with the mashed avocado, yogurt and chopped coriander.

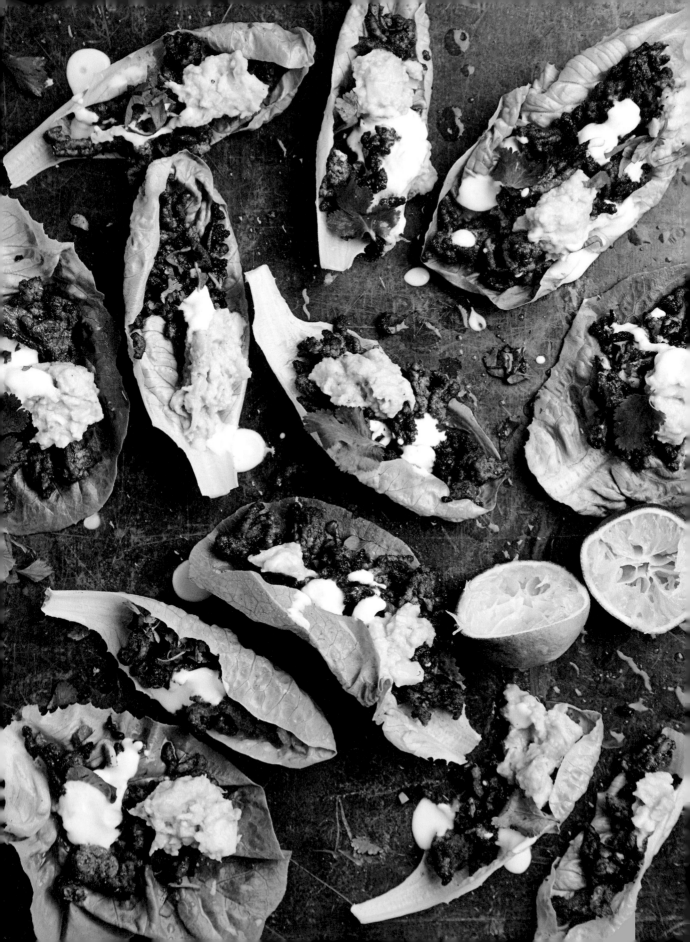

FISH

It's incredibly easy to make a quick fish supper. Pan-fry a fish fillet (you can buy them frozen to make life even simpler) or bake it in a parcel in the oven (page 117). Fill the rest of your plate with a pile of garlicky greens from the chapter starting on page 56. Dinner in a flash – done.

HOW TO COOK FISH

Cooking fish well is much easier than people think. The key is not to overcook it – serve it as soon as it is out of the oven and still deliciously tender. Fish is best eaten as fresh as possible, on the day it is bought. Timing depends on the thickness of the fillet: sea bass or bream fillets, for example, will cook in around 7 minutes whereas salmon fillets will take nearer 15 minutes. Pan-fried fish gives you a crispy skin and flavoursome, basted flesh, however I favour the healthier (and simpler) methods, such as baking and steaming.

BAKING

Simply baked fish, drizzled with olive oil and lemon (similar to the Tray Baked Salmon, Sweet Potato & Broccoli recipe on page 124) is a quick and easy method. Encasing the fish in foil or baking parchment retains more moisture and flavour (see Cod Parcels with Tomato, Olives, Capers & Rocket on page 117). This method is particularly good for thicker fillets like salmon, cod, trout, haddock and monkfish.

STEAMING

This is a great and healthy way to cook fish, retaining the moisture through the steam rather than any added oil or butter. I like to place the fish on a small piece of baking parchment inside the steamer to stop the skin sticking and to avoid messy washing up.

FAT (G): 23.2
PROTEIN (G): 30
SUGAR (G): 1.1
FIBRE (G): 1.1
CALORIES: 337
SERVES: 2

A lovely, light and zesty way to prepare salmon. Like fish cakes, but minus the stodgy addition of potato or breadcrumbs. Serve with the Broccoli & Courgette Salad with Peanut Dressing (see page 60).

SALMON & GINGER BURGERS

2 salmon fillets, skinned
4 spring onions, roughly chopped
2.5cm piece of root ginger, peeled and
    finely chopped
1 garlic clove, roughly chopped
½ small bunch of coriander (10–15g)
finely grated zest and juice of 1 unwaxed lime
salt and pepper
1 tbsp sesame oil
1 tbsp olive oil, plus more for your hands

Put all the ingredients except the olive oil into a food processor and pulse until roughly broken up (you don't want it to break down to a complete paste).

Shape into 2 burgers with your hands, rubbing a little oil on your palms first to make this less messy.

Heat the oil in a frying pan and gently fry the burgers for 3–4 minutes on each side.

FAT (G): 11.9
PROTEIN (G): 37
SUGAR (G): 4.9
FIBRE (G): 3.2
CALORIES: 295
SERVES: 2

The punchy Mediterranean flavours here pair perfectly with the delicate, sweet cod. You can make these parcels up to a day in advance and just bake them when you're ready to eat.

COD PARCELS WITH TOMATO, OLIVES, CAPERS & ROCKET

2 tomatoes, roughly chopped
50g pitted black olives, roughly chopped
1 heaped tsp capers, chopped
2 garlic cloves, chopped
finely grated zest and juice of 1 unwaxed lemon
15g flat-leaf parsley, chopped
1 tbsp olive oil, plus more for the fish
salt and pepper
50g rocket
2 skinless cod loins

"Baking fish in parcels keeps it moist, as well as infusing it with any flavours you add to the parcel. You can cook any fish fillets this way – just adjust the time depending on the thickness of the fish. Try adding one of the sauces on page 92."

Preheat the oven to 180°C/gas mark 4.

In a small bowl, mix together all the ingredients (including the 1 tbsp of oil) apart from the rocket and cod. Season well with salt and pepper.

Take a good length of foil or baking parchment (enough to wrap the cod and vegetables) and lay it over a baking tray. Place the rocket in the centre of the foil/paper, top with the tomato and olive mixture and lay the cod loins on top. Season the fish well with salt and pepper and drizzle with olive oil. Bring the edges of the foil/paper together, squeezing and folding them to create a sealed parcel.

Bake in the oven for 10–12 minutes.

Carefully unfold the parcels and serve with the juices and vegetables spooned over the fish.

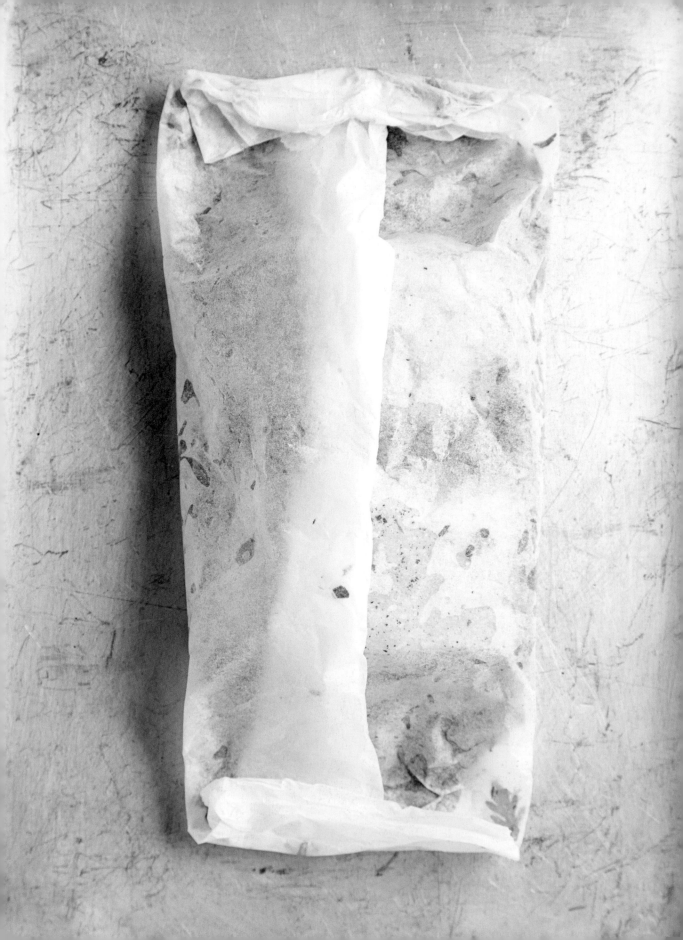

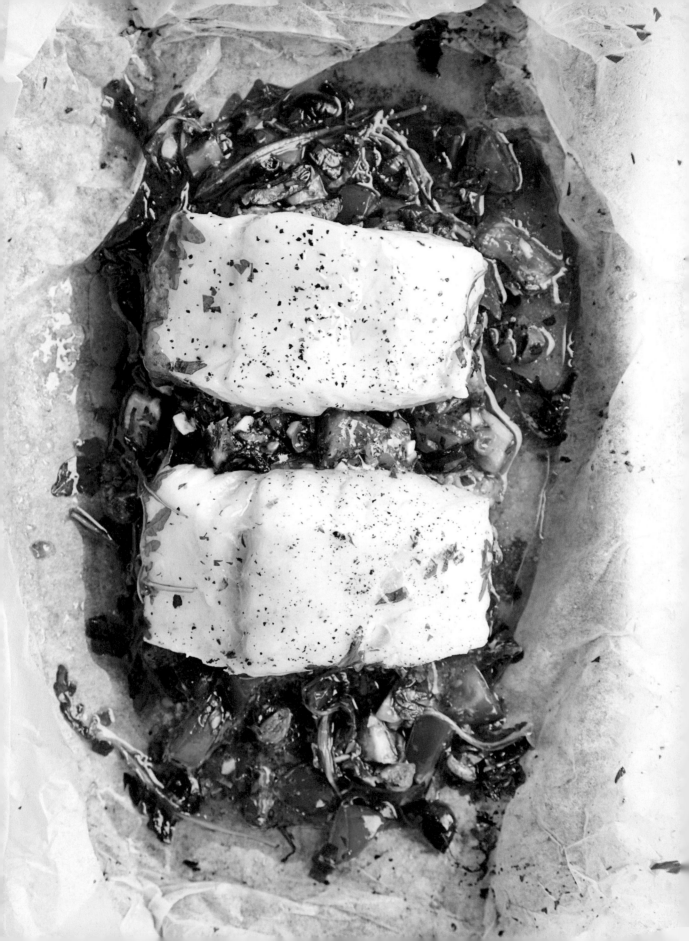

FAT (G): 7.7
PROTEIN (G): 34.2
SUGAR (G): 10.3
FIBRE (G): 8.6
CALORIES: 312
SERVES: 2

A vibrant one-pan dish, fresh and light enough for a summer supper but equally comforting in midwinter. Great for feeding a crowd, too, as it is easily multiplied. Serve with the Avocado, Fennel & Asparagus Salad (see page 64).

MEDITERRANEAN PRAWN STEW

2 tsp olive oil
1 small onion, chopped
1 fennel bulb, roughly chopped
4 garlic cloves, sliced
½–1 red chilli (depending on how spicy you like it), sliced
5 large tomatoes (about 500g), roughly chopped
splash of white wine
100ml fish or vegetable stock
125g white fish (I like coley, pollock or cod), cut into bite-sized pieces
125g raw prawns
finely grated zest and juice of 1 unwaxed lemon
small bunch of basil leaves, chopped
small bunch of flat-leaf parsley leaves, chopped

Heat the oil in a wide-based pan over a medium heat, add the onion and sauté for 5 minutes until soft. Add the fennel and sauté for a further 5 minutes. Add the garlic, chilli and tomatoes with the wine and increase the heat, mixing everything together. Cook until the wine has evaporated. Next, pour in the stock and reduce the heat to a light simmer. Cover and leave to cook for 10–15 minutes.

Add the fish and prawns to the pan and simmer for 3–4 minutes until just cooked (adding a splash more water if needed). Finally, add the lemon zest, juice and the herbs and serve.

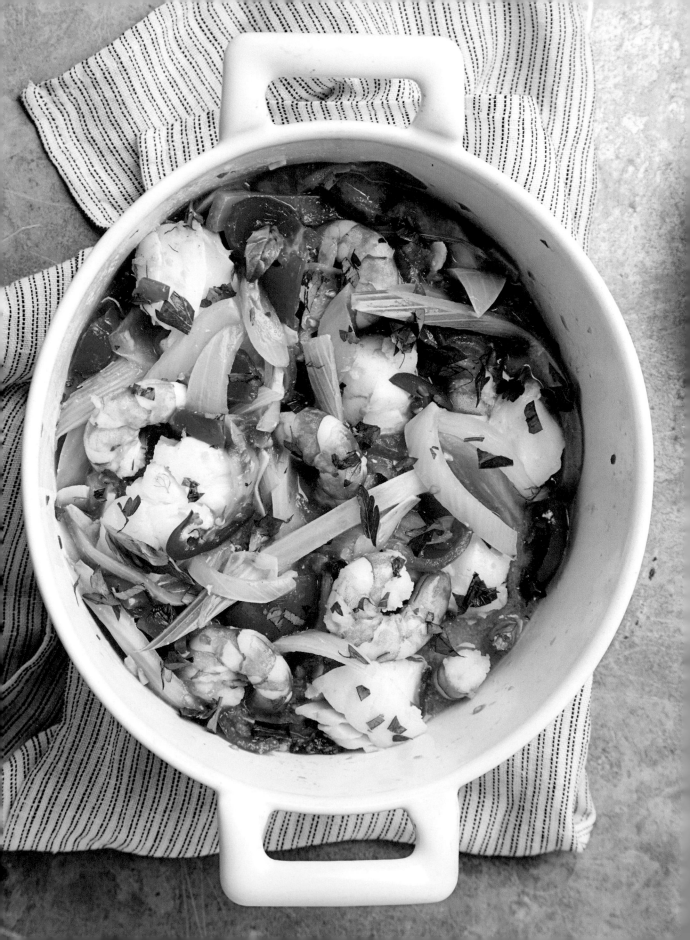

FAT (G): 42.9
PROTEIN (G): 22.7
SUGAR (G): 19.1
FIBRE (G): 10
CALORIES: 638
SERVES: 2

I love the sweetness of mango against the sharp, tangy Asian flavours and kick of chilli in this dish. This is a delicious, balanced bowl of food and great for a packed lunch, too.

PRAWN & MANGO NOODLE SALAD

For the salad
drizzle of olive oil
2 garlic cloves, sliced
165g raw prawns
100g rice noodles
1 avocado, peeled, stoned and chopped into cubes
1 mango, chopped into cubes

For the dressing
1 red chilli, chopped
10g coriander leaves, chopped
10g mint leaves, chopped
finely grated zest and juice of 1 unwaxed lime
1 tsp Dijon mustard
2 tbsp olive oil
1 tsp honey
2–3 drops of fish sauce

Heat the oil in a pan over a low heat and sauté the garlic for a minute or so. Add the prawns and cook for another 2–3 minutes until they are cooked through. Set aside to cool.

Place the noodles in a heatproof bowl, pour over freshly boiled water, cover with a plate and leave for 2 minutes, or until the noodles are soft. Drain and rinse well under cold water, drizzling with a little oil to stop from sticking.

For the dressing, whisk all the ingredients together in a small bowl or mug.

To assemble the salad, mix the avocado, mango and cooled prawns together, then stir through the noodles. Add the dressing to the bowl and mix well so that everything is nicely coated in those punchy flavours. Divide between 2 bowls and serve.

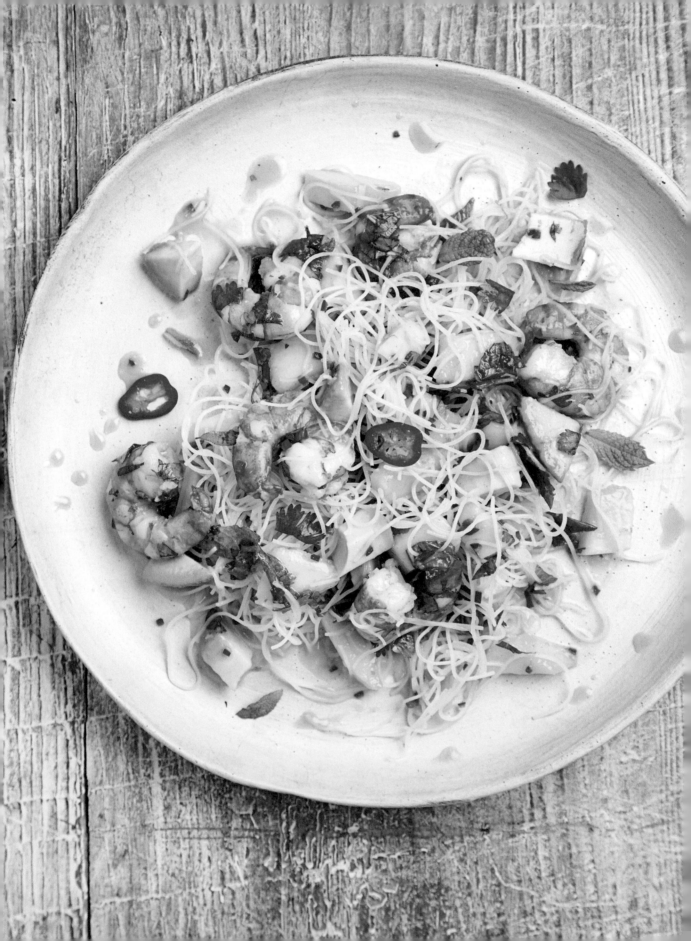

FAT (G): 23.7
PROTEIN (G): 32.5
SUGAR (G): 6.5
FIBRE (G): 4.2
CALORIES: 406
SERVES: 2

A colourful one-pan supper and great to prepare ahead, too: bake the potatoes and tomatoes, leave to cool, then top with the Tenderstem and salmon, cover with cling film and put in the fridge until you're ready to cook.

TRAY BAKED SALMON, SWEET POTATO & BROCCOLI

1 sweet potato, peeled and thinly sliced
100g cherry tomatoes
2 tbsp olive oil
salt and pepper
125g Tenderstem broccoli
2 salmon fillets
finely grated zest and juice of 1 unwaxed lemon
Salsa Verde (see page 92), to serve (optional)

Preheat the oven to 180°C/gas mark 4.

Lay the sweet potato discs in an ovenproof dish (large enough to fit the vegetables and salmon in). Put the tomatoes on top and drizzle with 1 tbsp of the olive oil, season well with salt and pepper and roast in the oven for 30 minutes.

Meanwhile, blanch the Tenderstem broccoli (for just 1 minute) in a pan of boiling water, then drain.

Remove the potatoes and tomatoes from the oven. Lay the broccoli and salmon on top, next to the tomatoes. Drizzle well with the remaining olive oil, lemon zest and juice and return to the oven for a further 12–15 minutes until the fish is just cooked.

Serve with Salsa Verde, if you like.

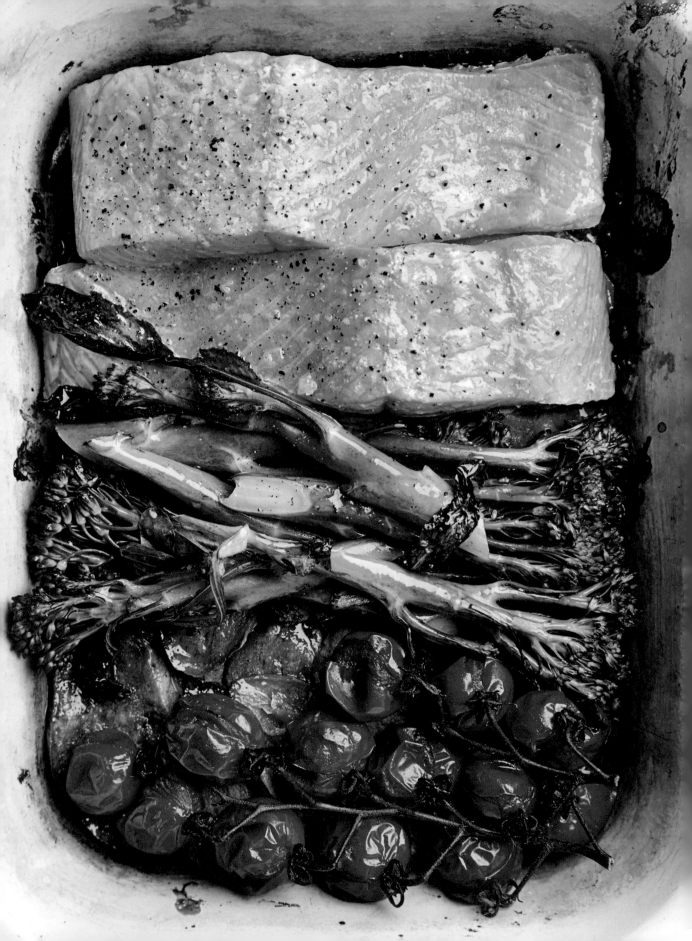

FAT (G): 23.2
PROTEIN (G): 30
SUGAR (G): 1.1
FIBRE (G): 1.1
CALORIES: 337
SERVES: 2

Sweetcorn fritters are quick and easy to make with storecupboard ingredients and a real hit with children, too. Delicious with the smoked salmon and the subtle spice of turmeric here.

CORN FRITTERS WITH SMOKED SALMON & TURMERIC YOGURT

250g sweetcorn (drained weight)
2 eggs
50g self-raising flour
salt and pepper
1 tbsp olive oil
1 tsp ground turmeric
100g natural yogurt
100g smoked salmon
30g rocket
½ small bunch of coriander, chopped
1 lemon, cut into wedges

Preheat the oven to 120°C/gas mark ½.

In a small bowl, combine the sweetcorn, eggs and flour and season well with salt and pepper.

Heat the olive oil in a frying pan, fry spoonfuls of the batter for 2 minutes each side, then transfer to a plate and keep warm in the low oven while you cook the rest.

In a bowl, mix the turmeric and yogurt together. Top the sweetcorn fritters with smoked salmon, a dollop of the turmeric yogurt and rocket, and sprinkle with the chopped coriander. Serve with the lemon wedges.

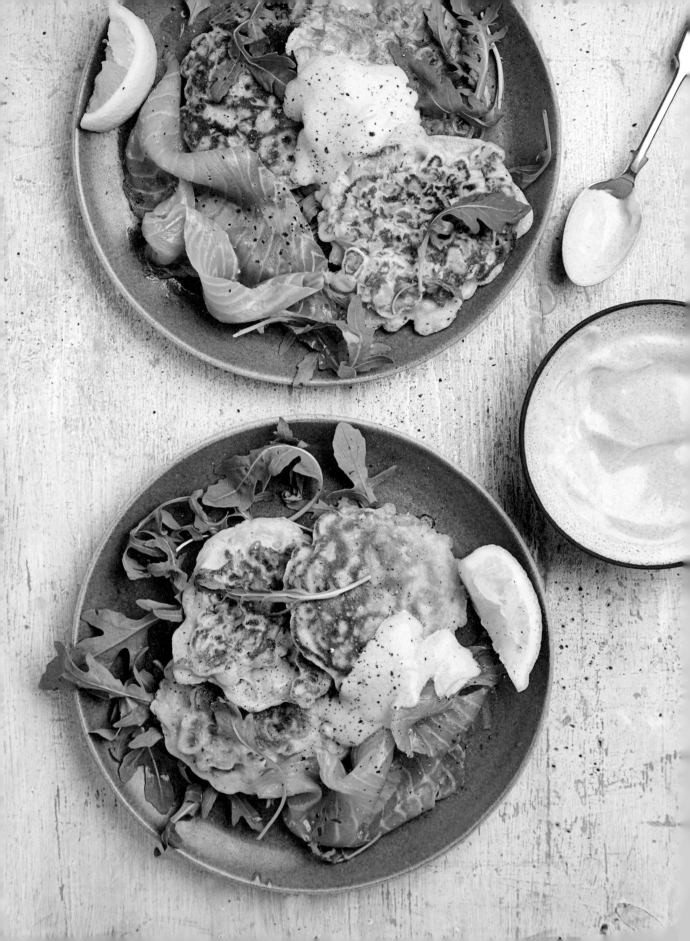

FAT (G): 55.9
PROTEIN (G): 7.1
SUGAR (G): 11.8
FIBRE (G): 7.3
CALORIES: 587
SERVES: 2

A light, zingy curry packed full of flavour. This is such a versatile recipe; add whatever meat, fish or vegetables you have in your fridge to the curry base (onion, garlic, chilli, spices and coconut milk) for a quick but impressive dinner.

COCONUT & TURMERIC FISH CURRY

1 tbsp coconut or sunflower oil
½ onion, finely chopped
½–1 red chilli (depending on how hot you like it), chopped
2 garlic cloves, finely chopped
1 heaped tsp ground turmeric
½ tsp garam masala
10 small dried curry leaves (if you can't get these, up the garam masala by ½ tsp)
400g can of coconut milk
150ml fish or vegetable stock
250g firm white fish (I like cod or monkfish), cut into chunks
1 small carrot, cut into matchsticks
1 small courgette, shaved into ribbons using a potato peeler
juice of 1 lime
salt and pepper
1 small bunch of coriander, chopped (optional)

Heat the oil in a pan and sauté the onion for 5 minutes, until translucent. Add the chilli, garlic, turmeric, garam masala and curry leaves (if using) and let all the flavours cook together for another 2–3 minutes, stirring regularly to ensure it doesn't catch.

Pour in the coconut milk and stock and simmer for 15 minutes. Reduce the heat to barely simmering, add the fish and vegetables and cook for another 3–4 minutes until the fish is just cooked and the vegetables are still nice and crunchy. Season well with salt and pepper. Squeeze over the lime juice, sprinkle with coriander, if you like, and serve with brown rice.

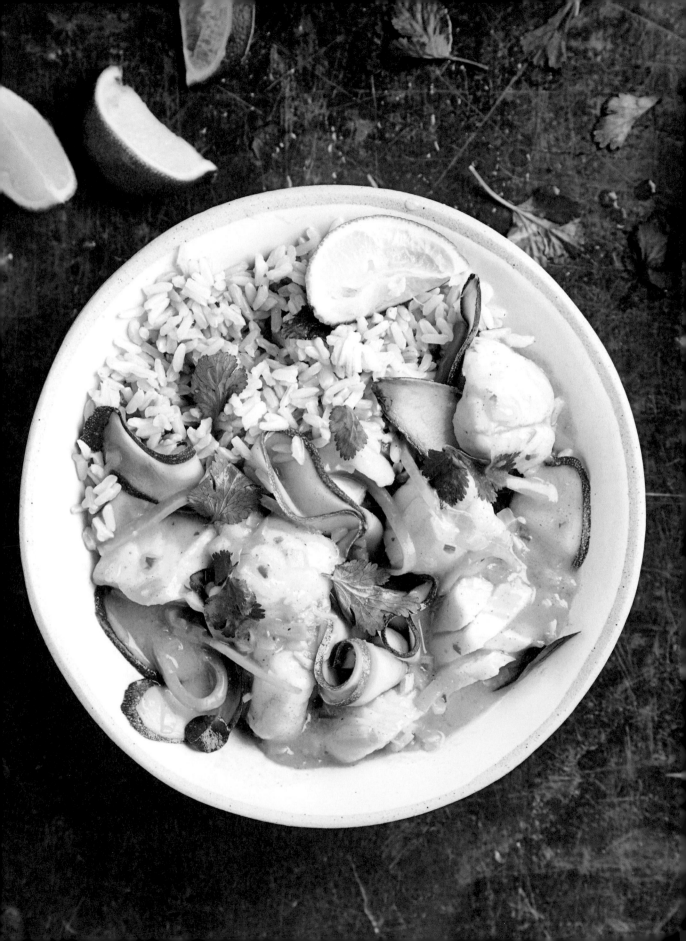

FAT (G): 21
PROTEIN (G): 28.1
SUGAR (G): 8.3
FIBRE (G): 8.4
CALORIES: 402
SERVES: 2

A slightly lighter take on a traditional fish pie, but still extremely comforting. Serve with a crunchy green salad or a big pile of steamed greens and you get a really good hit of nutrients from the trio of vegetables and the omega-packed fish.

FISH PIE WITH PEA & PARSNIP MASH

2 parsnips (about 200g), roughly chopped
125g petits pois
15g unsalted butter
4 spring onions, sliced
10g plain flour
2 tsp white wine vinegar
250ml fish or vegetable stock
25g crème fraîche
1 tsp wholegrain mustard
salt and pepper
200g mixed fish (use a fish pie mix, or I like equal amounts of salmon and smoked haddock)
150g spinach
1 tbsp olive oil
splash of milk (optional)

Preheat the oven to 180°C/gas mark 4.

Steam the parsnips over simmering water for 20–30 minutes until soft, adding the peas for the final 5 minutes. Drain and set aside.

Melt the butter in a saucepan and slowly sauté the spring onions for 5–10 minutes, until just starting to caramelize. Add the flour and mix well to create a paste. Pour in the vinegar and stir well. Next, pour in half the stock, keeping stirring really well over the heat; don't worry if it looks lumpy at first, it will gradually become a smooth sauce. Add the rest of the stock and continue to stir. Add the crème fraîche and mustard and season with salt and pepper to taste.

Add the fish and cook over a low heat for another 2–3 minutes until just cooked.

Wilt the spinach in a separate pan with a little boiling water, rinse under cold water and drain really well, squeezing out as much water as you can. Roughly chop the spinach and stir through the fish mix.

Pour into a small ovenproof dish and set aside whilst you finish the topping. Put the parsnips and petits pois into a food processor with the olive oil, season well with salt and pepper and pulse until smooth; alternatively mash roughly with a potato masher. Add a splash of water or milk to loosen up, if necessary.

Spoon the mash over the fish mixture and bake in the oven for 20–25 minutes, until the top is crispy and golden.

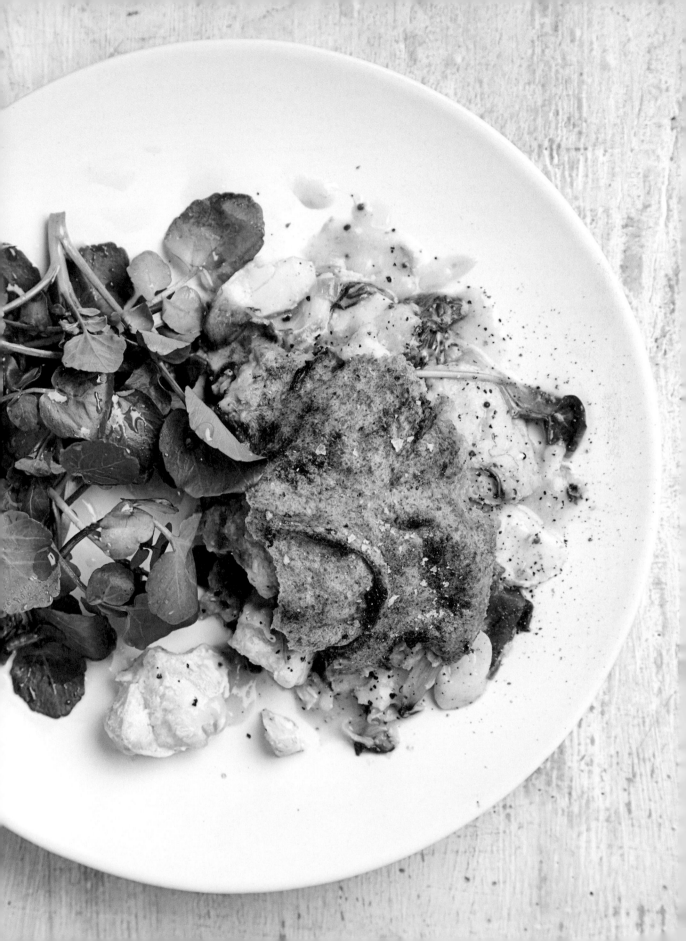

FAT (G): 42.2
PROTEIN (G): 22.9
SUGAR (G): 22.1
FIBRE (G): 7
CALORIES: 601
SERVES: 2

Smoked mackerel is a wonderful ingredient for a quick and easy dinner. The oily fish is rich in omega-3s and pairs perfectly with the sweet tang of citrus and earthy depth of beetroot. This is a lovely lunch or light supper; it also travels well as a packed lunch if you keep the dressing separate.

SMOKED MACKEREL, BEETROOT & ORANGE SALAD

For the salad
½ small butternut squash (about 200g),
   cut into half moon shapes (no need to peel)
1 tbsp olive oil
salt and pepper
50g mixed salad leaves
2 small cooked beetroot, cut into wedges
2 smoked mackerel fillets, skinned and broken
   into bite-sized pieces
1 orange, skin removed and cut into segments

For the dressing
10g dill, coarse stalks removed and chopped
3 tbsp olive oil
juice of 1 lemon
squeeze of honey
pinch of salt

Preheat the oven to 180°C/gas mark 4.

Put the squash into a roasting tin, drizzle with the olive oil and season well with salt and pepper. Roast for 20–30 minutes until soft, then leave to cool.

To make the dressing, simply whisk all the ingredients together in a small bowl or mug.

To assemble the salad, lay the salad leaves on a serving platter, top with the beetroot and squash and finally the mackerel pieces and orange segments. Drizzle with the dressing and serve.

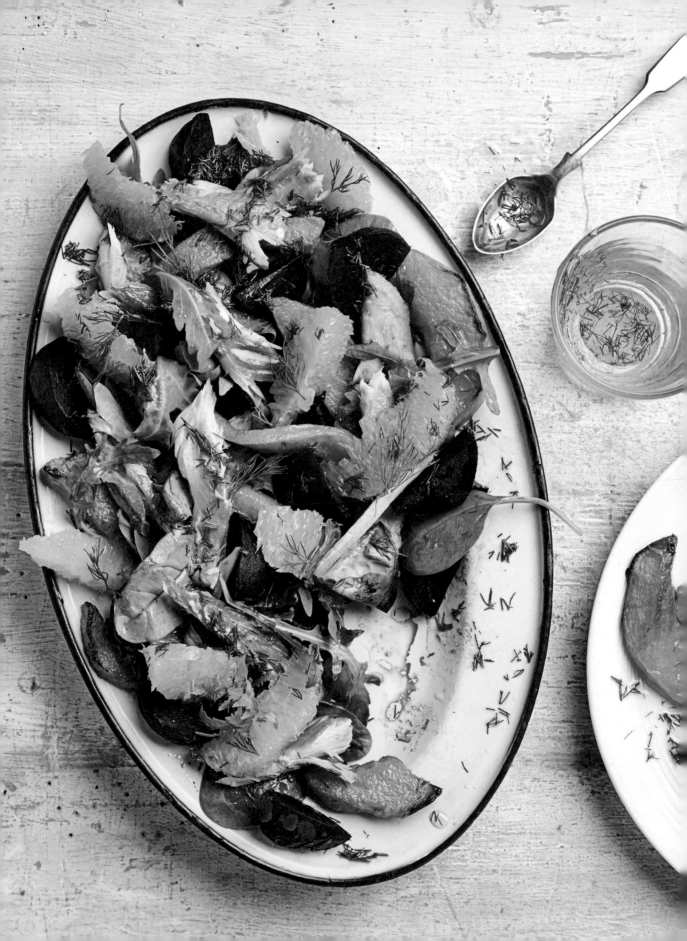

FAT (G): 22
PROTEIN (G): 37.8
SUGAR (G): 8.2
FIBRE (G): 7.8
CALORIES: 651
SERVES: 2

This is a wonderfully balanced bowl of food, both nutritionally and in terms of flavour and texture. Feel free to cook your tuna for longer if you don't like it rare. For extra spice, add a sliced chilli, or serve with wasabi.

JAPANESE RICE & TUNA BOWL

For the rice bowl
140g brown rice
salt
2 tbsp sesame seeds
200g tuna steak
1 tbsp sunflower or sesame oil
5 spring onions, sliced
2.5cm piece of root ginger, peeled and finely
    chopped or grated
100g petits pois
4 radishes, topped, tailed and sliced

For the dressing
finely grated zest and juice of 1 unwaxed lime
1 tbsp rice wine vinegar, or ½ tbsp white
    wine vinegar
2 tsp maple syrup, or honey
1 tbsp soy sauce

Cook the brown rice in a large pan of salted boiling water for 25–30 minutes, or until tender but retaining a nutty bite. Drain and set aside.

Meanwhile, sprinkle the sesame seeds on a plate or board, lay the tuna on top and turn until each side is roughly coated in seeds.

Heat the oil in a frying pan over a high heat. Add the tuna to the pan and sear it on each side for 10–20 seconds. Remove the tuna from the pan and set aside (do not wash up the pan yet).

Next, make the dressing by mixing all the ingredients together in a small bowl or mug.

Put the pan back over the heat and sauté the spring onions and ginger for 2–3 minutes until soft. Add the peas and radishes to the pan and turn off the heat.

Next, add the cooked rice and dressing to the pan and stir everything together well over a low heat. While the rice and vegetables warm through, slice the tuna into strips about 5mm thick.

Divide the rice mixture between 2 bowls, top with the sliced tuna and serve immediately.

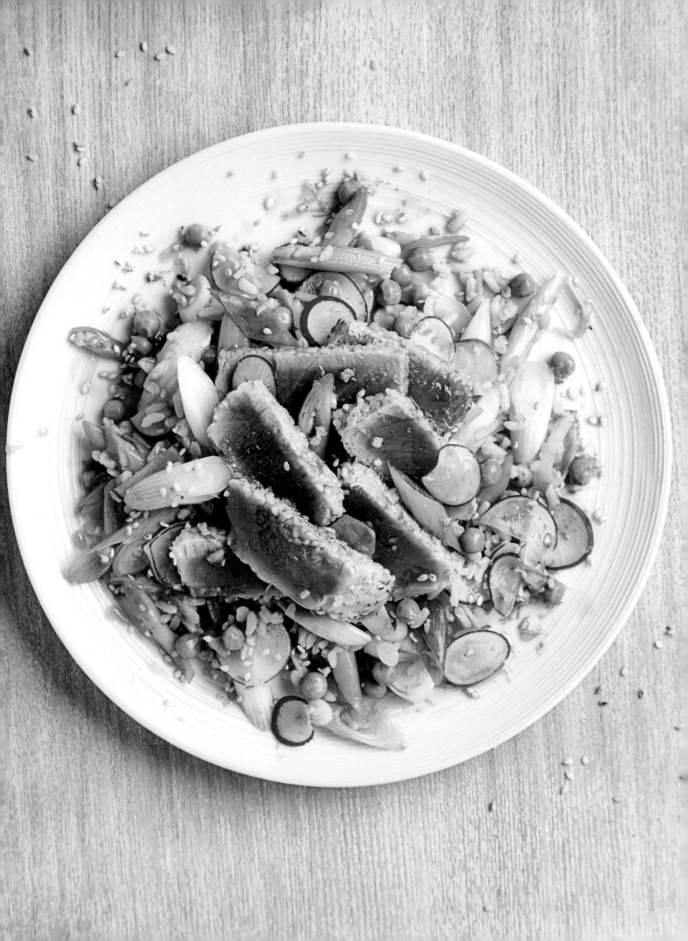

VEGETABLE MAINS

These recipes all suit vegetarians (just make sure
you buy vegetarian cheese where needed)
but you shouldn't rule out this chapter if you're
a meat eater. The dishes will fill you up and give you
an opportunity to branch out from your meat-and-veg routine.
Give them a try. You might find yourself embracing
part-time vegetarianism – especially useful if you can't
afford to buy the best-quality meat every day.

FAT (G): 18.9
PROTEIN (G): 35.7
SUGAR (G): 18.9
FIBRE (G): 34.6
CALORIES: 652
SERVES: 2

The carrots are the star of the show here; their caramelized sweetness works perfectly with the slightly tangy goat's cheese. The Puy lentils make it a filling but nutritious lunch.

ROAST CARROT, GOAT'S CHEESE & LENTIL SALAD

3 carrots (about 300g), quartered lengthways
3 garlic cloves, quartered
1 tbsp olive oil
1 tbsp honey
finely grated zest and juice of 1 unwaxed lime
200g cooked Puy lentils
salt and pepper
80g baby leaf salad
65g soft goat's cheese, crumbled
Tahini Dressing (see page 57), to serve

Preheat the oven to 160°C/gas mark 3.

Place the carrots, garlic, oil, honey, lime zest and juice into a baking tray and roughly mix to coat the carrots in all of the lovely flavours. Cover with foil and roast in the oven for 45 minutes or until the carrots are soft. Remove from the oven, pour the lentils into the baking tray with the carrots and mix well to coat in the sticky roasting juices. Season very well with salt and pepper.

Arrange the salad leaves on a serving plate, pour over the lentils and carrots and crumble over the goat's cheese. Serve with Tahini Dressing.

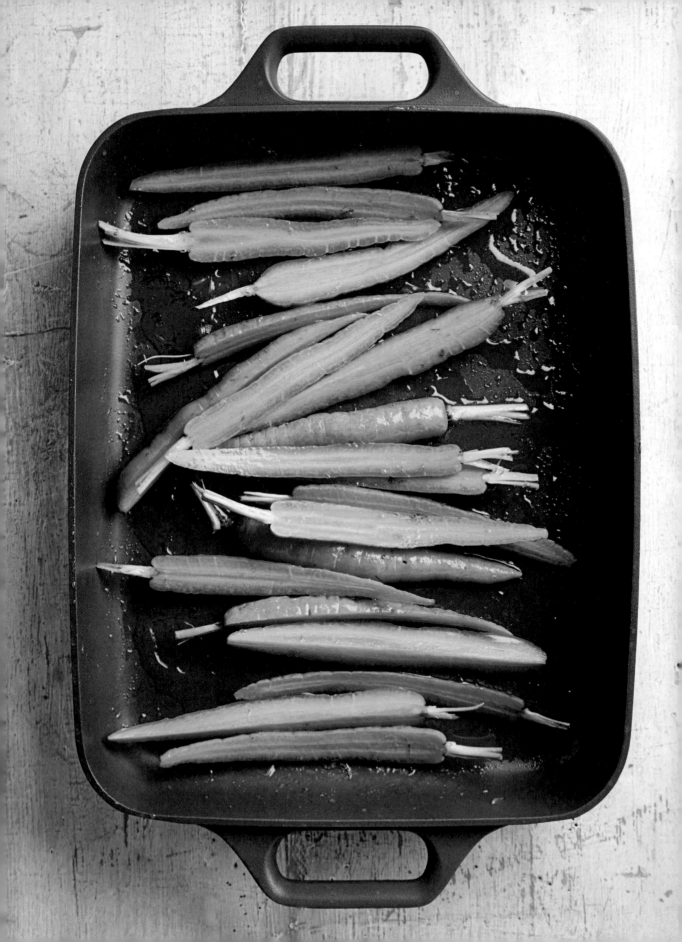

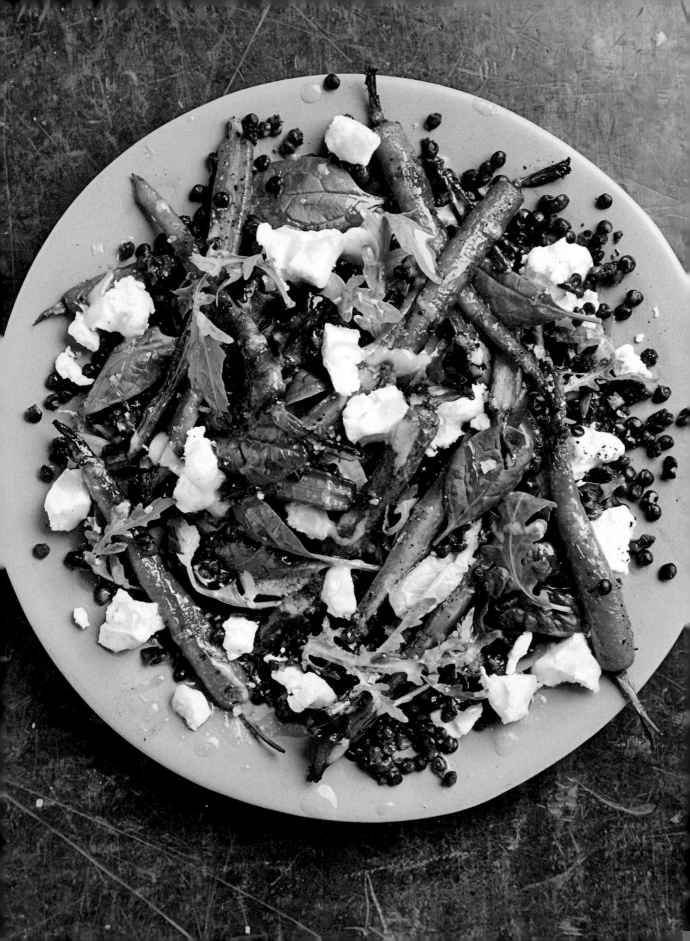

FAT (G): 37.9
PROTEIN (G): 15.5
SUGAR (G): 4.7
FIBRE (G): 3.8
CALORIES: 439
SERVES: 2

Whole Portobello mushrooms make a substantial vegetarian main course. The salty tang from the feta is lovely with the fragrant pesto.

PESTO & FETA PORTOBELLO MUSHROOMS

30g basil
50g kale, coarse stalks removed
2 garlic cloves
2 tbsp olive oil
50g nuts (almonds, cashews or pine nuts)
100g feta
2 Portobello mushrooms
pepper

Preheat the oven to 180°C/gas mark 4.

Place the basil, kale, garlic, olive oil, nuts and half the feta into a food processor with 2 tbsp of water. Process until you have a smooth pesto. Turn the mushrooms stalk side up and cut the stalks out with a small knife. Spoon the pesto into each mushroom, dividing it equally between them. Top with the remaining 50g of feta and season with pepper (they will be salty enough from the feta so no need for more salt).

Bake in the oven for 25–30 minutes, then serve.

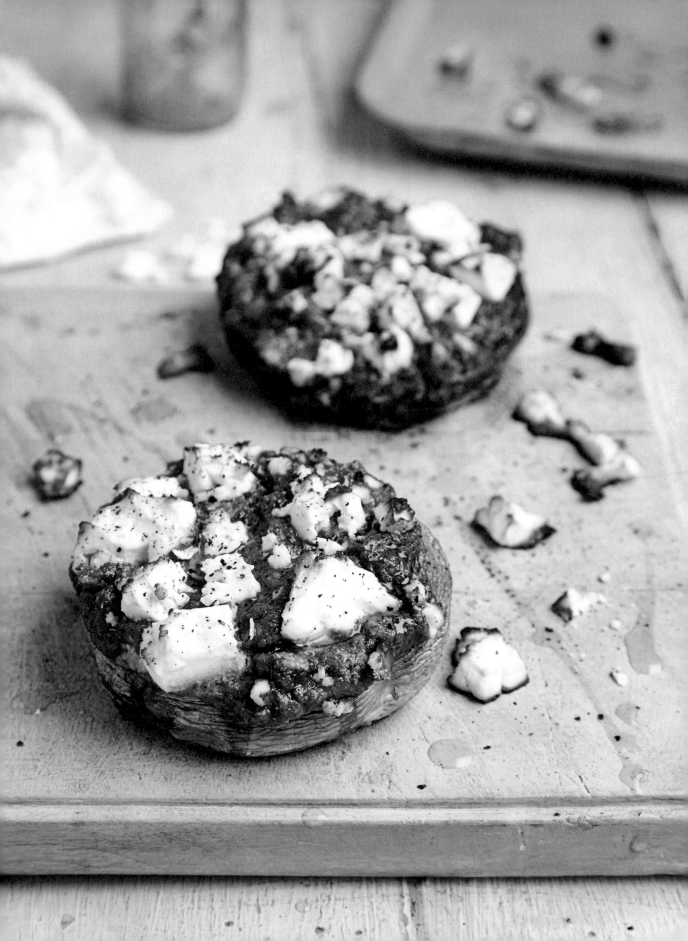

FAT (G): 15.4
PROTEIN (G): 10.5
SUGAR (G): 16.3
FIBRE (G): 13.5
CALORIES: 276
SERVES: 2

This is a wonderful main dish, best
served with a crunchy green salad.
It also goes perfectly with some simply
grilled chicken or fish.

AUBERGINE & COURGETTE GRATIN

1 aubergine, sliced lengthways
1 tbsp olive oil, plus more for drizzling
salt and pepper
½ red onion, chopped
2 garlic cloves, sliced
425g tomatoes (about 6), roughly chopped
small bunch of basil leaves, roughly chopped
1 courgette, sliced lengthways
20g Parmesan, finely grated
15g pine nuts

Preheat the oven to 180°C/gas mark 4.

Lay the aubergine slices in a baking tray, drizzle with
olive oil and season well with salt and pepper. Roast
in the oven for 15 minutes until the aubergine is soft.

Meanwhile, heat the 1 tbsp olive oil in a pan, add the
onion and sauté for 5 minutes until soft. Add the
garlic and tomatoes and cook for a further 5 minutes.
Add the basil to the pan and simmer for 10–15
minutes, until the tomatoes break down and you
have a sauce.

Spoon a layer of the tomato sauce into a small
ovenproof dish, follow with a layer of aubergine and
courgette and then some more sauce. Repeat the
layers, finishing with a layer of the tomato sauce. Top
with the Parmesan and pine nuts. Bake in the oven
for 25 minutes, until the top is golden.

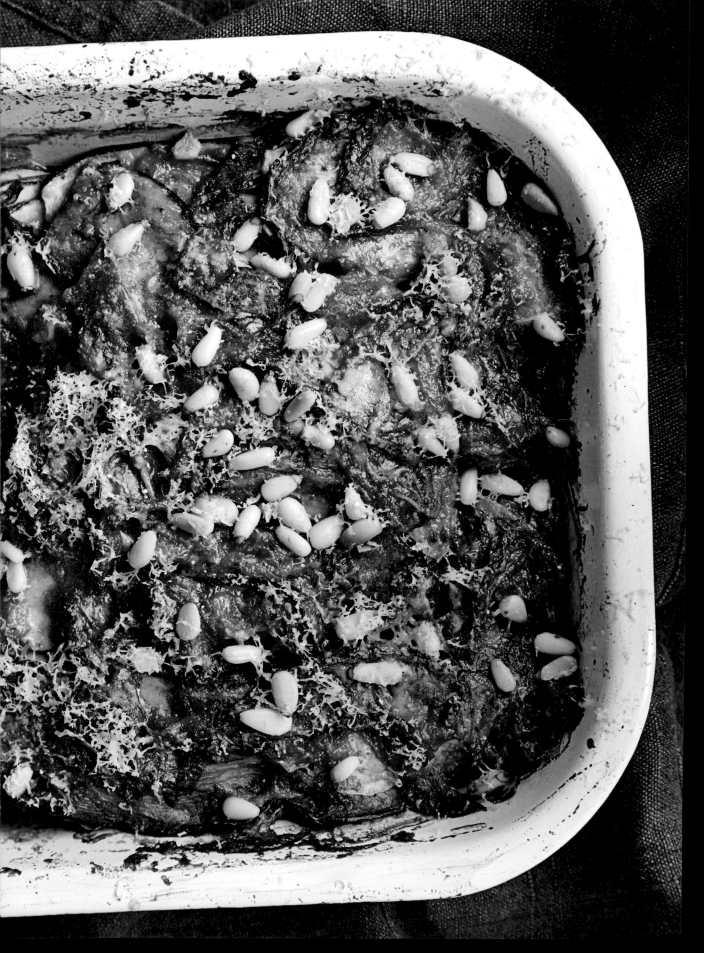

FAT (G): 56.4
PROTEIN (G): 19.9
SUGAR (G): 15.9
FIBRE (G): 22.9
CALORIES: 808
SERVES: 2

Dhal is my go-to comfort dish – lightly spiced, warming and nutritious – perfect after a long day. Serve with a big dollop of yogurt. Leftovers keep well in the fridge for lunch the next day.

SWEET POTATO & SPINACH DHAL

1 tbsp sunflower oil
½ onion, chopped
3 garlic cloves, chopped
1 heaped tsp ground turmeric
1 tsp garam masala
85g red lentils
1 sweet potato (about 200g), peeled and cubed
400g can of coconut milk
salt and pepper
juice of 1 lime
100g spinach
1 red chilli, sliced (optional)

Heat the oil in a saucepan and sauté the onion for 5 minutes, until soft. Add the garlic, turmeric and garam masala and cook for a further minute. Add the lentils, potato and coconut milk and simmer for 35–40 minutes, until the lentils are cooked and breaking down and the sweet potato is soft. Keep an eye on it as it cooks, stirring occasionally and adding a splash of water if it looks a little dry.

Season well with salt, pepper and the lime juice, Remove from the heat, add the spinach and put a lid on the pan to allow the leaves to wilt. Stir the wilted spinach through and serve with the chilli sprinkled over, if you want.

FAT (G): 26.9
PROTEIN (G): 21
SUGAR (G): 1.6
FIBRE (G): 0.9
CALORIES: 353
SERVES: 2

FAT (G): 36.2
PROTEIN (G): 16.6
SUGAR (G): 11.5
FIBRE (G): 12.4
CALORIES: 478
SERVES: 2

Eggs make a wonderful protein-packed alternative to meat or fish. Here are two of my favourite ways to bake them: delicious, quick and easy one-pan suppers.

BAKED EGGS

KALE AND GOAT'S CHEESE

125g kale, coarse stalks removed
1 tbsp olive oil
75g soft goat's cheese
4 eggs
salt and pepper

Preheat the oven to 180°C/gas mark 4.

Steam the kale over simmering water for 2 minutes, until just wilted. Put it in an ovenproof dish, drizzle with the olive oil and crumble over the goat's cheese. Carefully crack the eggs over the top: this is easiest if you make slight indents in the kale with the back of the spoon first for the eggs to nestle in.

Season well with salt and pepper and bake in the oven for 8–15 minutes, or until the whites are just set but the yolks are soft.

TOMATO AND AVOCADO

1 tbsp olive oil
1 small onion, chopped
2 garlic cloves, sliced
1 red pepper, sliced
1 tsp paprika
400g can of chopped tomatoes
salt and pepper
1 avocado, peeled, stoned and sliced
4 eggs
25g coriander, chopped

Preheat the oven to 180°C/gas mark 4.

Heat the oil in a saucepan and sauté the onion for 5 minutes until soft, then add the garlic, red pepper and paprika and cook for a further 2 minutes before adding the chopped tomatoes and seasoning well with salt and pepper. Simmer gently for 10 minutes.

Spoon the tomato sauce into an ovenproof dish, lay the sliced avocado on top and carefully crack the eggs over and in between the avocado slices. Bake in the oven for 8–15 minutes, or until the whites are just set but the yolks are still soft. Sprinkle with the coriander and serve.

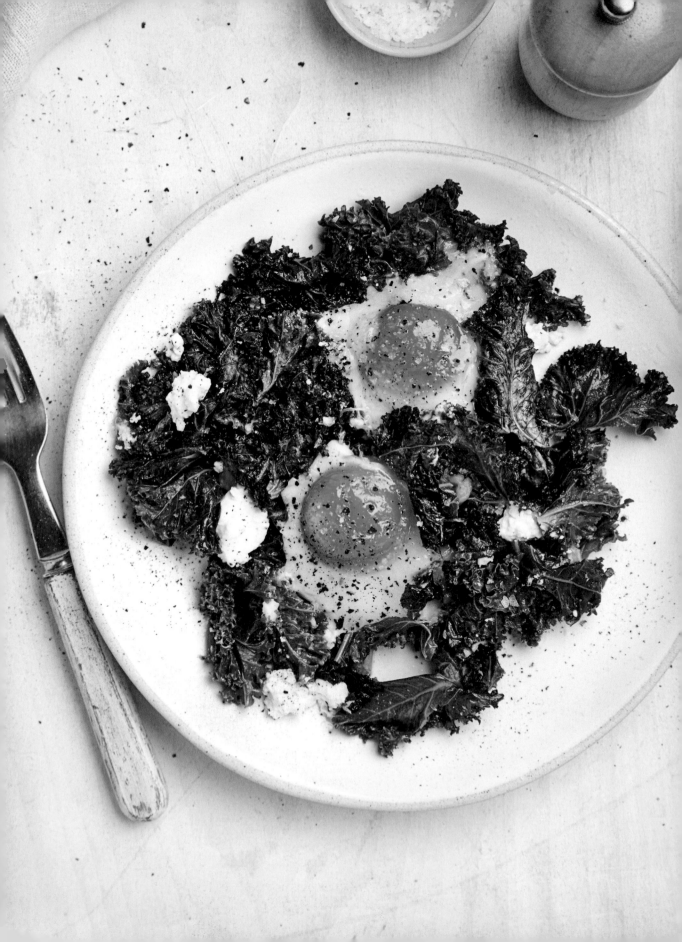

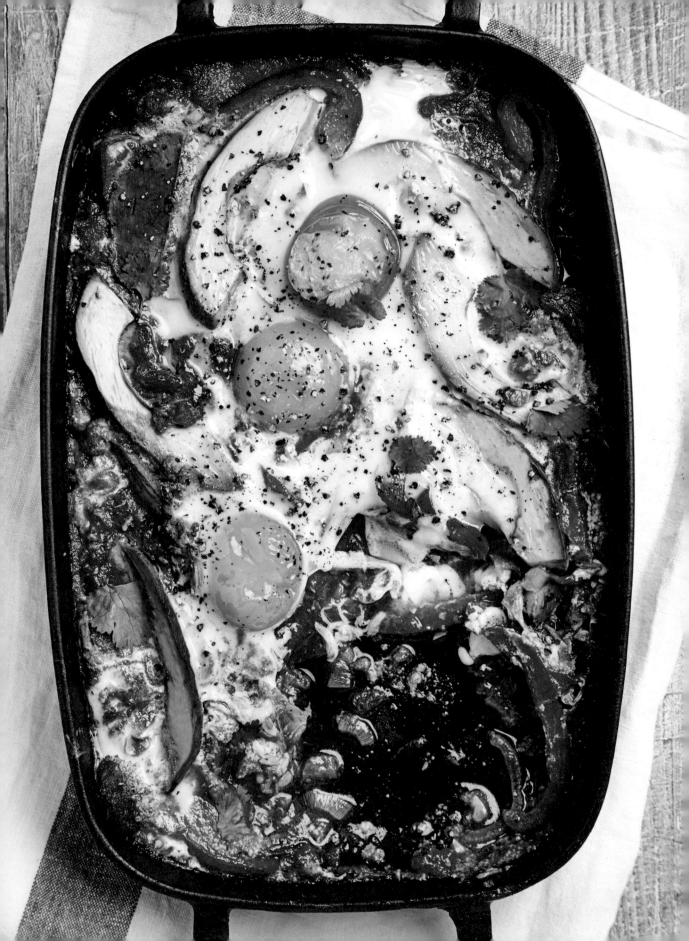

FAT (G): 11.9
PROTEIN (G): 11.9
SUGAR (G): 5.1
FIBRE (G): 6.5
CALORIES: 351
SERVES: 2

A lighter version of a traditional risotto, but equally creamy and comforting. Quinoa is also protein-rich, so this is a great vegetarian option. Serve with the Garlicky Green Veg (see page 68).

COURGETTE, ROCKET & GOAT'S CHEESE QUINOA RISOTTO

1 leek, sliced
2 garlic cloves, sliced
1 tbsp olive oil
120g quinoa
1 tbsp cider vinegar
600ml vegetable stock
finely grated zest and juice of 1 unwaxed lemon
65g soft goat's cheese
30g rocket, roughly chopped
1 courgette, grated

Sauté the leek and garlic in the oil over a medium heat for 5 minutes until soft. Tip in the quinoa and stir over the heat for a couple of minutes. Add the vinegar and cook until it has evaporated, then pour in the stock and bring to the boil. Simmer for 20–35 minutes (stirring occasionally) until most of the stock has been absorbed and you are left with a creamy consistency. If the quinoa looks like it's drying, just add a splash more water.

Reduce the heat to its lowest and add the lemon zest and juice, the goat's cheese, rocket and courgette. Mix everything together well until the cheese has melted and serve.

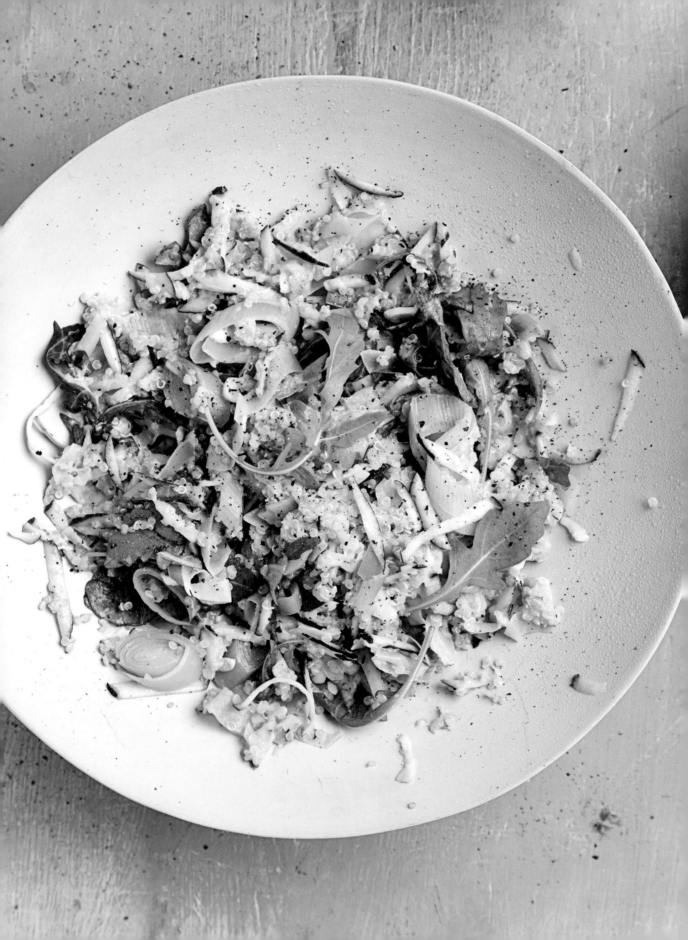

FAT (G): 2
PROTEIN (G): 5.5
SUGAR (G): 7.2
FIBRE (G): 3.4
CALORIES: 146
SERVES: 2

A quick and nutritious dinner. The spiced broth is perfect for when you're feeling under the weather, or have a cold coming on!

MUSHROOM & PAK CHOI PHO

1 litre vegetable stock
3 star anise
1 cinnamon stick
2 garlic cloves, chopped
2.5cm piece of root ginger, peeled and sliced into matchsticks
½–1 red chilli, chopped (depending on how hot you want it)
120g shiitake mushrooms, roughly chopped
100g rice or buckwheat noodles
1 bulb of pak choi, quartered
juice of 1 lime, plus lime wedges to serve
1 tsp honey
15g coriander, chopped

"Keep stock, spices and dried rice noodles in your storecupboard and then just add whatever vegetables you have in your fridge for the ultimate speedy supper when you're short on time."

First make the broth: heat the stock in a saucepan with the star anise, cinnamon, garlic, ginger and chilli. Simmer for 10 minutes to let the flavours infuse the broth.

Add the mushrooms to the pan and cook for 5 minutes. Add the noodles and pak choi and cook for a further 2–3 minutes (or as stated on the noodle packet instructions). Reduce the heat to its lowest and add the lime juice and honey. Either fish out the star anise and cinnamon sticks at this stage, or just watch out for them when eating! Divide between 2 bowls and serve with chopped coriander sprinkled over and lime wedges on the side.

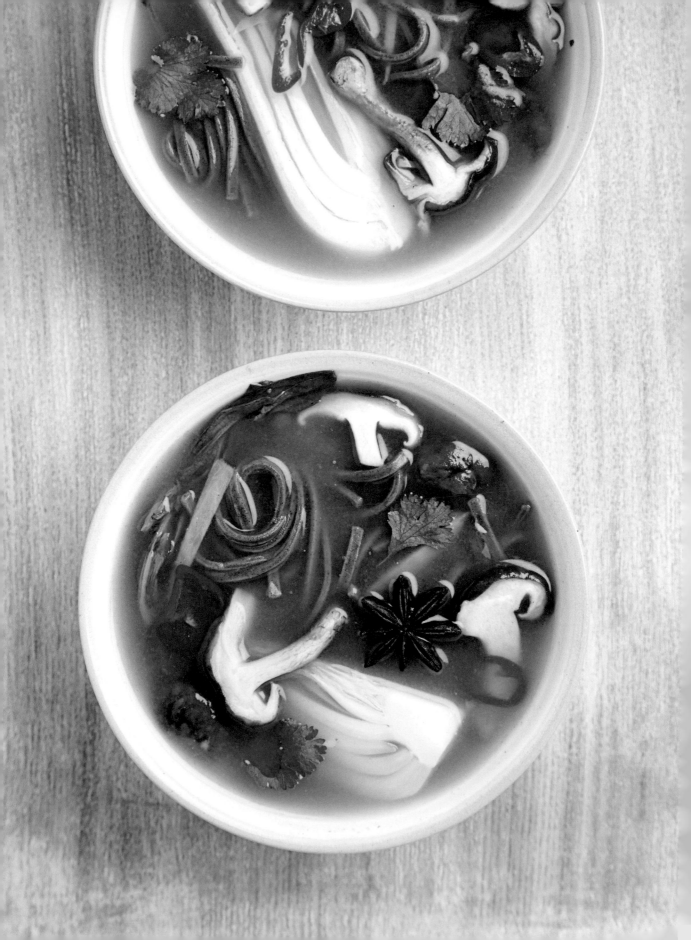

FAT (G): 56.5
PROTEIN (G): 25.3
SUGAR (G): 36.9
FIBRE (G): 24.1
CALORIES: 812
SERVES: 2

A whole roast cauliflower is a really impressive main course and a wonderful way to use an often-overlooked vegetable. Serve with the Avocado, Fennel & Asparagus Salad (see page 64).

ROAST CAULIFLOWER WITH ROMESCO

1 large cauliflower (750–800g) or 2 small
1 red onion, sliced
100g sun-dried tomatoes, chopped
1 tbsp olive oil
1 x quantity Romesco (see page 92)
200ml vegetable stock
salt and pepper
1 tbsp flaked almonds
10g flat-leaf parsley leaves, chopped

Preheat the oven to 180°C/gas mark 4.

Pull or cut the leaves away from the cauliflower and discard. Trim the stem and slice the cauliflower (if large) in half lengthways, through the stalk. Lay the onion and sun-dried tomatoes in a roasting tray and drizzle with the olive oil. Rub the Romesco sauce all over the cauliflower halves and place on top of the onions and tomatoes. Pour over the stock and season well with salt and pepper.

Cover with foil and roast for 40 minutes. Remove the foil and baste the cauliflower well with the stock. Sprinkle over the flaked almonds, then return the tray to the oven for a further 20 minutes, or until the cauliflower is tender.

Serve with the juices, onion and sun-dried tomatoes spooned over and parsley sprinkled over the top. Delicious served with garlicky yogurt or Tahini Dressing (see page 57).

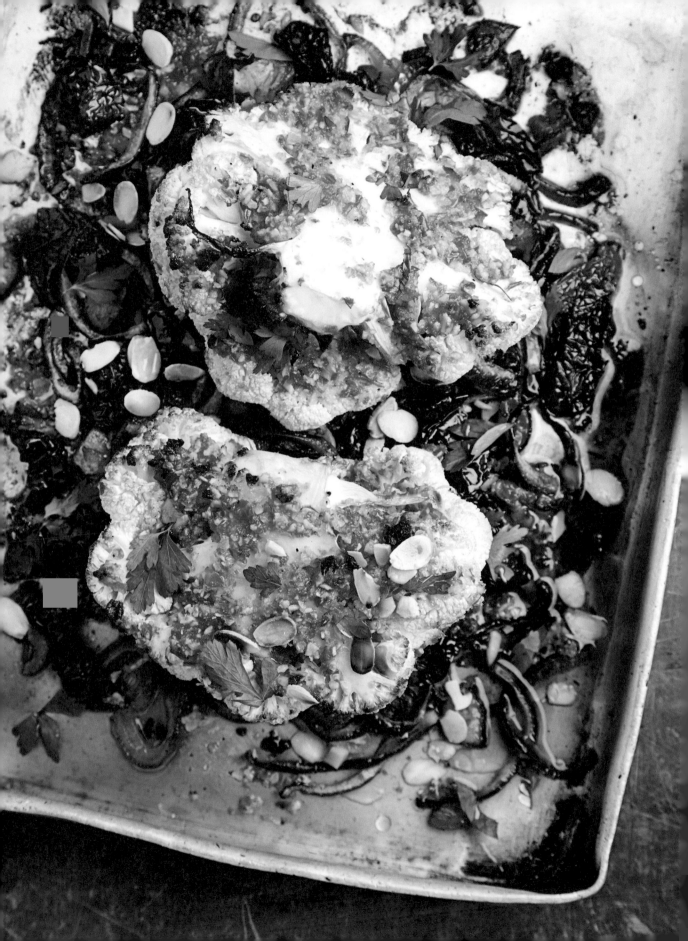

FAT (G): 57.1
PROTEIN (G): 14.1
SUGAR (G): 1.7
FIBRE (G): 8.1
CALORIES: 523
SERVES: 2

It may sound mad to massage the kale leaves, but it actually really works: the leaves wilt in the oil and lemon juice and become tender enough to eat raw.

KALE, AVOCADO & SOFT EGG SALAD

2 eggs
125g kale, stalks removed, leaves roughly chopped
juice of 1 lemon
pinch of salt
2 tbsp olive oil
1 avocado, peeled, stoned and sliced
20g Parmesan, shaved with a potato peeler
20g pine nuts, toasted in a dry pan
Dijon Dressing (see page 57), to serve

Boil a small pan of water, add the eggs and simmer for 7 minutes to soft boil them, then drain and leave to cool in cold water.

Meanwhile, put the kale, lemon juice, salt and oil into a bowl and massage the leaves with your hands for 5–10 minutes until they are wilted, soft and dark green. Arrange the kale on a serving dish.

Carefully remove the shells from the eggs and cut them into quarters. Arrange over the kale with the avocado, shaved Parmesan and pine nuts. Serve with Dijon Dressing.

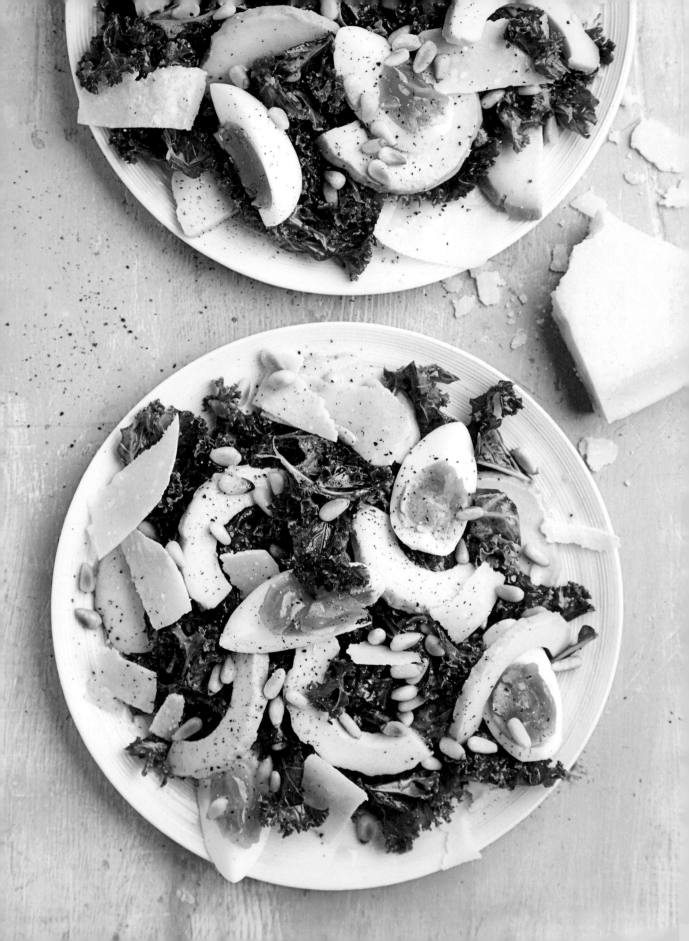

FAT (G): 28.2
PROTEIN (G): 7.7
SUGAR (G): 5.2
FIBRE (G): 11
CALORIES: 345
SERVES: 2

The avocado in this recipe is used instead of potato to give a thick and creamy texture.

SUPER GREEN SOUP

1 tbsp olive oil
½ small onion, chopped
2 garlic cloves, sliced
½ head of broccoli, finely chopped (stalk included)
750ml hot vegetable stock, plus more if needed (optional)
85g spinach
1 avocado, peeled and stoned
finely grated zest and juice of 1 unwaxed lemon
salt and pepper

Heat the oil in a pan and sauté the onion for 5 minutes until soft. Add the garlic and sauté for a further couple of minutes before adding the broccoli and stock and bringing everything to the boil. Simmer for another 5 minutes until the broccoli is cooked.

Add the spinach to the pan, put the lid on, turn off the heat and leave it to wilt for a couple of minutes. Add the avocado, lemon zest and juice and blend well in a food processor or with a hand-held blender, adding more stock or water if you prefer it thinner.

To serve, gently reheat and season well with salt and pepper to taste.

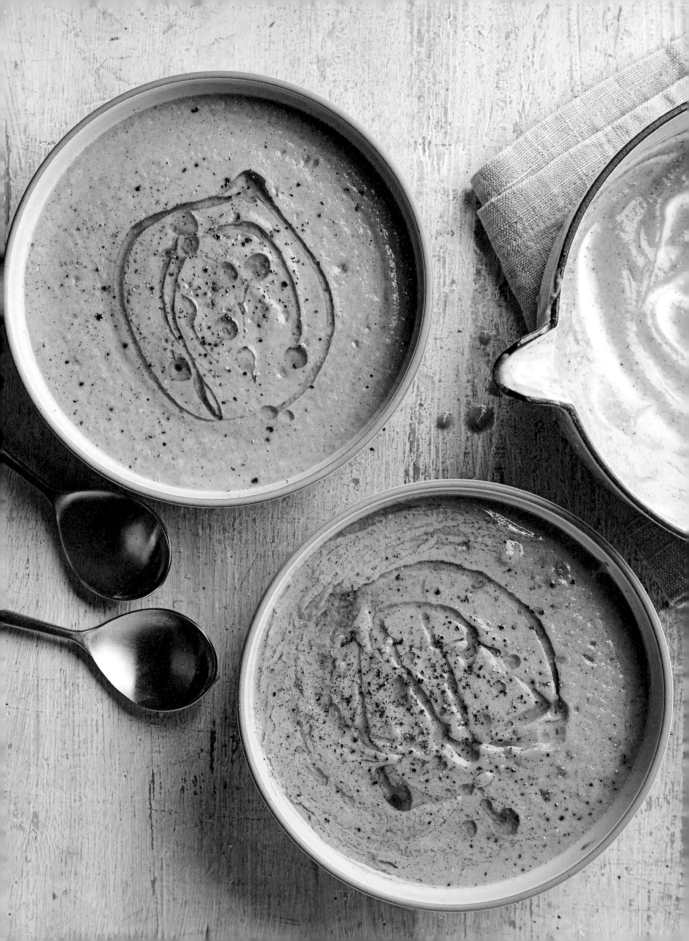

FAT (G): 8.7
PROTEIN (G): 4
SUGAR (G): 7.8
FIBRE (G): 5.3
CALORIES: 197
SERVES: 2

A vibrant, zesty and warming soup that keeps well in the fridge for a couple of days.

SQUASH, GINGER & LEMON SOUP

1 tbsp olive oil
½ onion, chopped
2 garlic cloves, sliced
½ small butternut squash, deseeded and roughly chopped (no need to peel)
1 carrot, roughly chopped
2.5cm piece of root ginger, peeled and roughly chopped
1 tsp ground turmeric
750ml vegetable stock
juice of 1 lemon

Heat the oil in a saucepan and sauté the onion for 5 minutes until soft. Add the garlic and cook for a further couple of minutes before adding the squash, carrot, ginger and turmeric.

Pour the stock over the vegetables and bring to the boil, then reduce the heat and simmer for 20 minutes until the vegetables are soft. Leave to cool slightly, before blitzing in a food processor or with a hand-held blender with the lemon juice, adding more stock or water if you prefer it thinner.

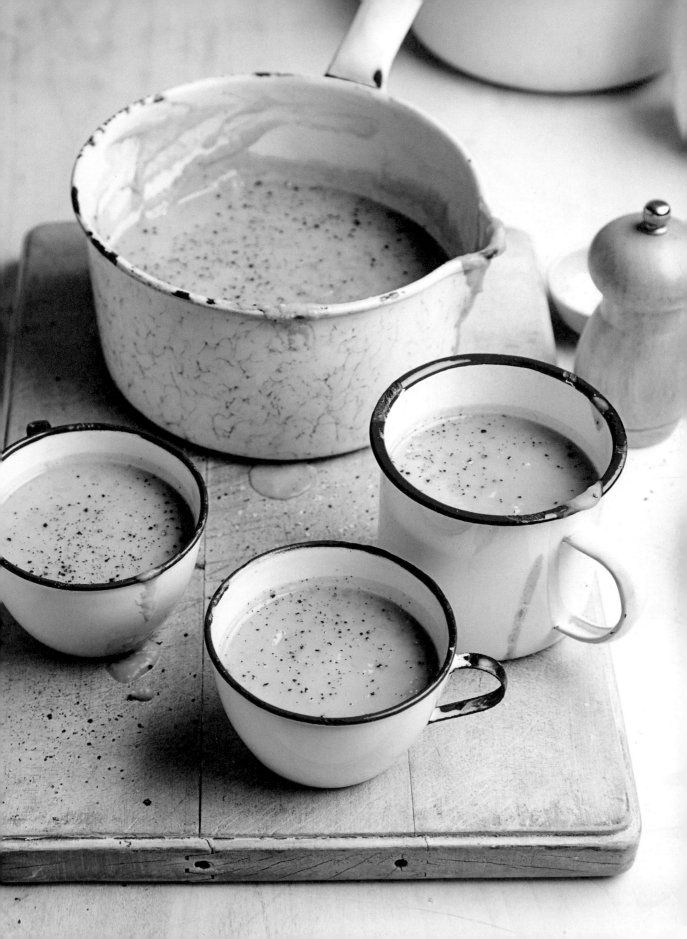

PUDDINGS

Georgie wouldn't let me just have the pudding
section say: "chop up a piece of fruit".
She's right. Some nights you need pudding.
Especially if you're entertaining.
Or dining with your special person.
Or alone in front of the TV.

FAT (G): 17.4
PROTEIN (G): 7
SUGAR (G): 20
FIBRE (G): 6.2
CALORIES: 319
SERVES: 2

A lovely weekend pudding, with just a little butter and honey to sweeten it, and no flour. It's a more virtuous version of a traditional crumble.

PLUM & BLUEBERRY CRUMBLE

500g plums (about 8), stoned and quartered
finely grated zest and juice of 1 unwaxed orange
1 tsp vanilla extract
35g plus 1 tbsp honey
100g oats
75g ground almonds
50g unsalted butter
1 tsp ground cinnamon
300g blueberries
35g flaked almonds
natural yogurt, to serve

Preheat the oven to 180°C/gas mark 4.

Place the plums in a baking dish with the juice and zest of the orange, the vanilla extract and 1 tbsp honey. Bake for 10 minutes. Meanwhile, combine the oats, ground almonds, butter, 35g honey and cinnamon in a bowl with your hands; it should stick together like a wet crumble.

Remove the plums from the oven and add the blueberries to the dish. Top the fruit with the crumble mixture, spooning it evenly over the berries and plums. Finally, sprinkle with the flaked almonds and return to the oven for 20–25 minutes. Serve with natural yogurt.

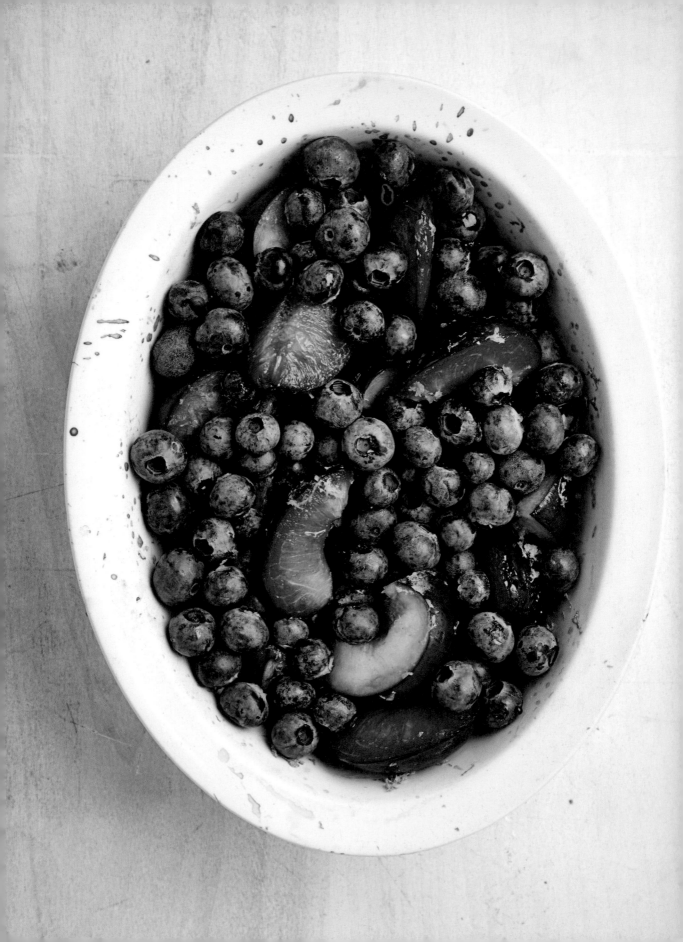

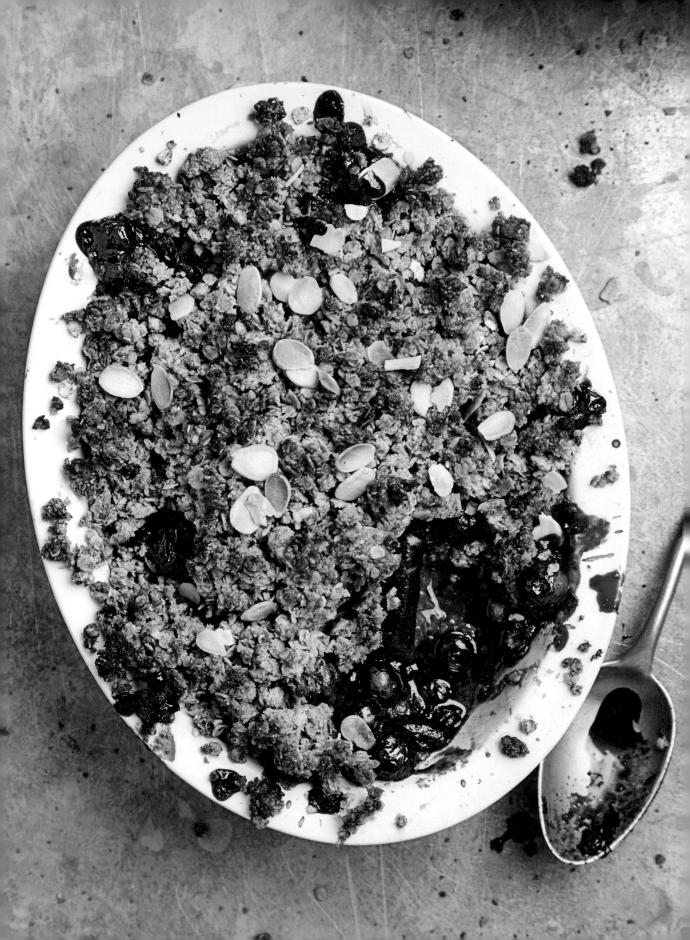

(CHOCOLATE) FAT (G): 0.7
PROTEIN (G): 1.8
SUGAR (G): 14.5
FIBRE (G): 3.9
CALORIES: 111
SERVES: 2

(SALTED PEANUT) FAT (G): 10.8
PROTEIN (G): 7.7
SUGAR (G): 18.1
FIBRE (G): 4.3
CALORIES: 240
SERVES: 2

(BERRY) FAT (G): 0.8
PROTEIN (G): 2.9
SUGAR (G): 18.3
FIBRE (G): 4.1
CALORIES: 140
SERVES: 2

This recipe may seem like a bizarre concept, but the frozen banana really does give a creamy, ice cream-like texture when blended in a food processor. Keep a stash of peeled bananas (take the time to do this, as it's a nightmare trying to peel them when frozen) in your freezer and whizz up a bowl when ice cream cravings get the better of you. Here are three of my favourite flavour combinations.

BANANA 'ICE CREAM'

Chocolate
2 bananas, peeled and frozen
1 tbsp cocoa powder

Salted peanut
2 bananas, peeled and frozen
40g peanut butter
pinch of salt
50g natural yogurt

Berry
2 bananas, peeled and frozen
60g frozen berries
50g natural yogurt

For any of these 3 flavours, the method is the same: place all the ingredients in the food processor and pulse until smooth. It may take a minute or so to reach a smooth consistency as the banana melts.

FAT (G): 13.3
PROTEIN (G): 8.1
SUGAR (G): 14.4
FIBRE (G): 5.3
CALORIES: 256
SERVES: 2

It's important to have some good snack ideas up your sleeve to steer you away from junk food when you're out and about. Make a batch of these at the weekend and they will keep really well in an airtight container in the fridge for the coming week. They also freeze well as individual bars and defrost quickly. The combination of dates, nuts and orange makes them the perfect afternoon pick-me-up.

ORANGE & ALMOND GRANOLA BARS

200g pitted dates
60ml warm water
125g peanut butter
150g oats
100g flaked almonds
20g sesame seeds
pinch of salt
finely grated zest of 1 unwaxed orange

Preheat the oven to 180°C/gas mark 4. Line a baking tin (approximately 20cm or 23cm square) with baking parchment.

Put the dates, water and peanut butter into a food processor and blend. Add the oats and pulse a couple of times, so the oats are still chunky but combined. Pour this mixture into a bowl, then add the flaked almonds, sesame seeds, salt and orange zest and mix well.

Spoon the mixture into the lined baking tray and flatten evenly with the back of the spoon (it should be 1–2cm thick).

Bake for 10–12 minutes until firm and golden. Leave to cool slightly in the tin for 10–15 minutes, then loosen the edges with a knife and cut into 10–12 bars while still slightly warm. Remove from the tin and leave to cool completely on a wire rack.

FAT (G): 5.5
PROTEIN (G): 8.8
SUGAR (G): 24
FIBRE (G): 3.4
CALORIES: 204
SERVES: 2

The soft, creamy ricotta pairs excellently with the sweet, sticky fruit and tangy citrus. Serve as pudding and eat the leftovers for breakfast. This recipe is perfect for using up under- or over-ripe fruit.

BAKED RICOTTA WITH PEACHES & FIGS

2 figs, halved
2 peaches, halved and stoned
½ tub of ricotta (125g)
drizzle of honey
1 tsp vanilla extract
finely grated zest and juice of 1 unwaxed lemon
1 tbsp flaked almonds

> "Baked fruit with a couple of extra ingredients is suddenly elevated to pudding-worthy status."

Preheat the oven to 180°C/gas mark 4.

Place the figs and peaches, cut sides up, in an ovenproof dish.

Using a teaspoon, dot the ricotta over the fruit evenly.

Drizzle over the honey, vanilla extract, lemon zest and juice.

Finally, sprinkle over the flaked almonds and bake for 30–40 minutes until the fruit is tender and golden.

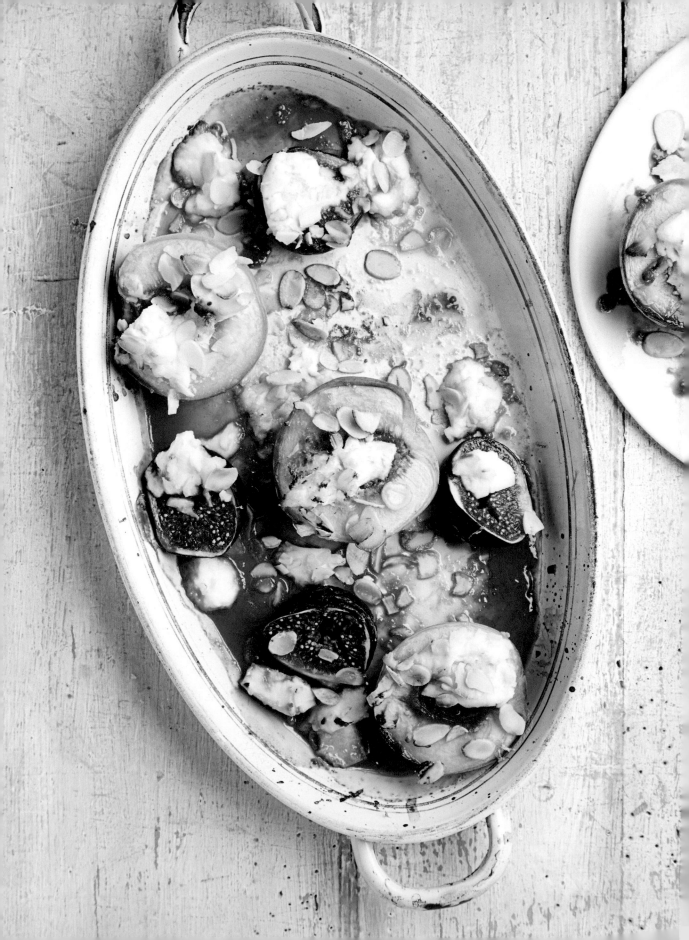

FAT (G): 0.7
PROTEIN (G): 1.5
SUGAR (G): 40.9
FIBRE (G): 7.5
CALORIES: 219
SERVES: 2

This is a more exciting fruit salad, perfect if you want to serve pudding to friends but stay away from anything naughty. The fragrant herbs and sweet berries are a lovely match for the tangy pineapple.

PINEAPPLE WITH SMASHED BASIL RASPBERRIES

1 pineapple, peeled, cored and cut into slices
125g raspberries
juice of 1 lime
2 tsp honey
leaves from ½ small bunch of mint, finely chopped
leaves from ½ small bunch of basil, finely chopped

Arrange the pineapple on a plate.

In a small bowl, roughly crush the raspberries with the back of a fork, add the lime juice, honey and herbs and stir well. Spoon the raspberry mixture over the top of the pineapple and serve.

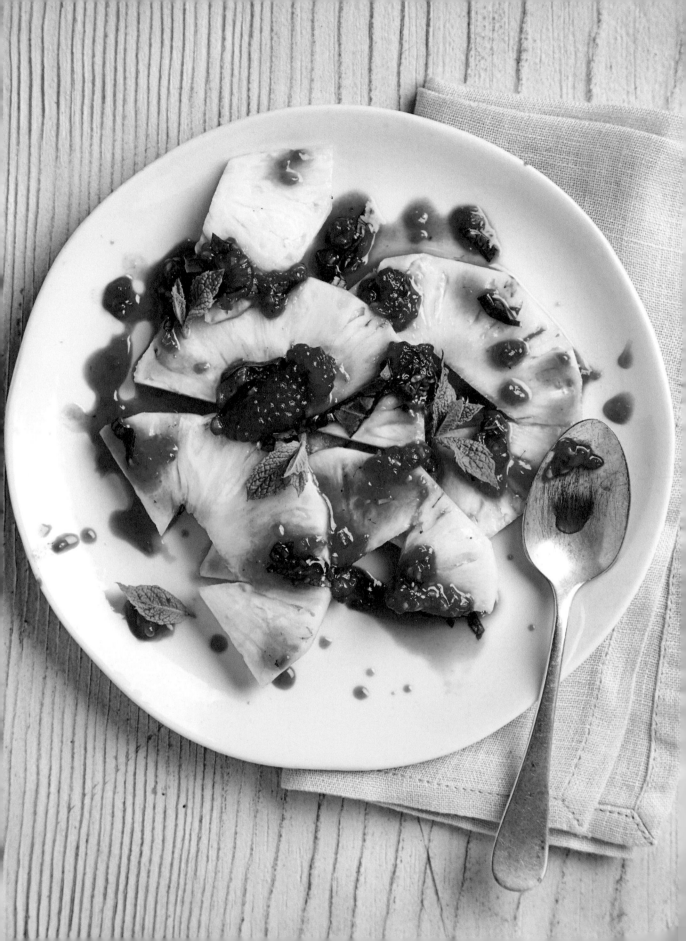

FAT (G): 0.5
PROTEIN (G): 1.7
SUGAR (G): 24.1
FIBRE (G): 5.1
CALORIES: 130
SERVES: 2

The pears in this recipe are poached in an aromatic hit of cardamom, cinnamon and citrus zest. Serve warm or cold with crème fraîche or yogurt.

CARDAMOM POACHED PEARS

900ml water
1 tbsp cardamom pods, roughly crushed
2 cinnamon sticks
1 tsp vanilla extract
2 tbsp honey
finely grated zest and juice of 1 unwaxed orange
finely grated zest and juice of 1 unwaxed lemon
2 pears, peeled but kept whole

Place all the ingredients into a small saucepan and bring to the boil. Reduce the heat to a simmer and cook for 15 minutes, or until the pears are tender but not too soft. Remove the pears from the poaching liquid and place in a serving bowl.

Increase the heat to a brisk boil and reduce the poaching liquid for about 15 minutes, until it is turning syrupy. Pour around half of it over the pears (or as much as desired, discard the rest).

Serve warm or cold.

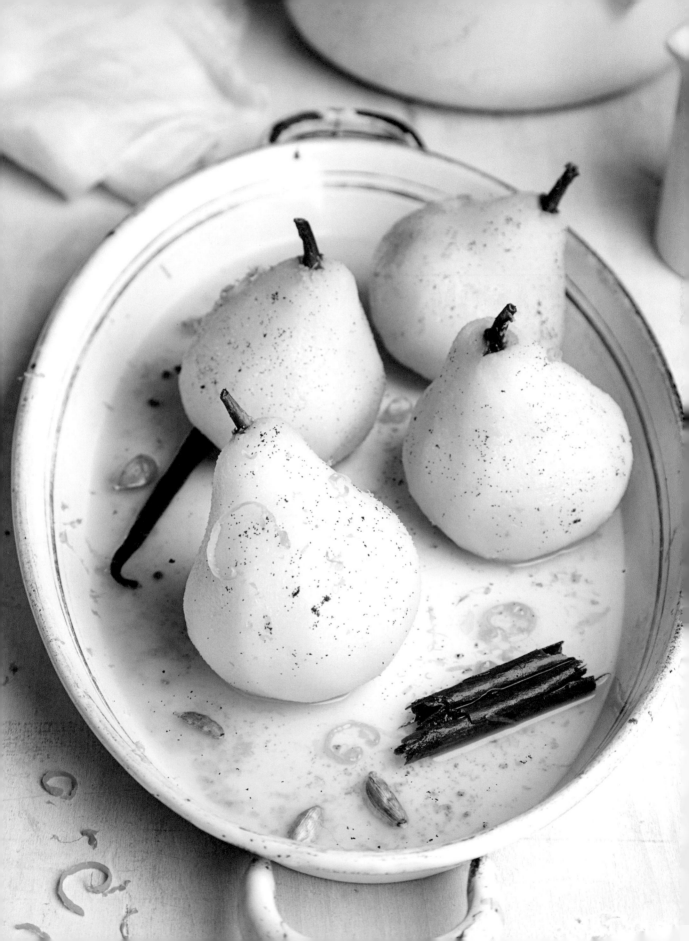

FAT (G): 26.9
PROTEIN (G): 7.3
SUGAR (G): 29.6
FIBRE (G): 4.5
CALORIES: 414
SERVES: 2

Serve these after your Spaghetti Carbonara on a cheat day (see page 105). Then get someone stronger than you to roll you to bed. Intensely rich and spoiling, and best served with cold cream or ice cream.

GOOEY CHOCOLATE POTS

125g dark chocolate
125g unsalted butter
4 eggs
100g caster sugar
35g self-raising flour
35g cocoa powder
pinch of salt
150g frozen mixed berries (I like the summer fruits packets from the supermarket)

> "This is not diet food. Everyone needs a fabulous chocolate pudding recipe up their sleeve for a special occasion."

Preheat the oven to 200°C/gas mark 6.

Melt the chocolate and butter in a saucepan over a low heat, then set aside to cool.

Crack the eggs into a bowl, add the sugar and mix well. Pour the cooled chocolate and butter mixture into the bowl with the sugar and eggs and mix together. Add the flour, cocoa powder and salt and mix.

Divide the frozen berries between 6 ramekins and pour the chocolate mixture on top.

Bake in the oven for 10–12 minutes until just set on top but still gooey in the middle.

Serve with cold cream, yogurt or ice cream.

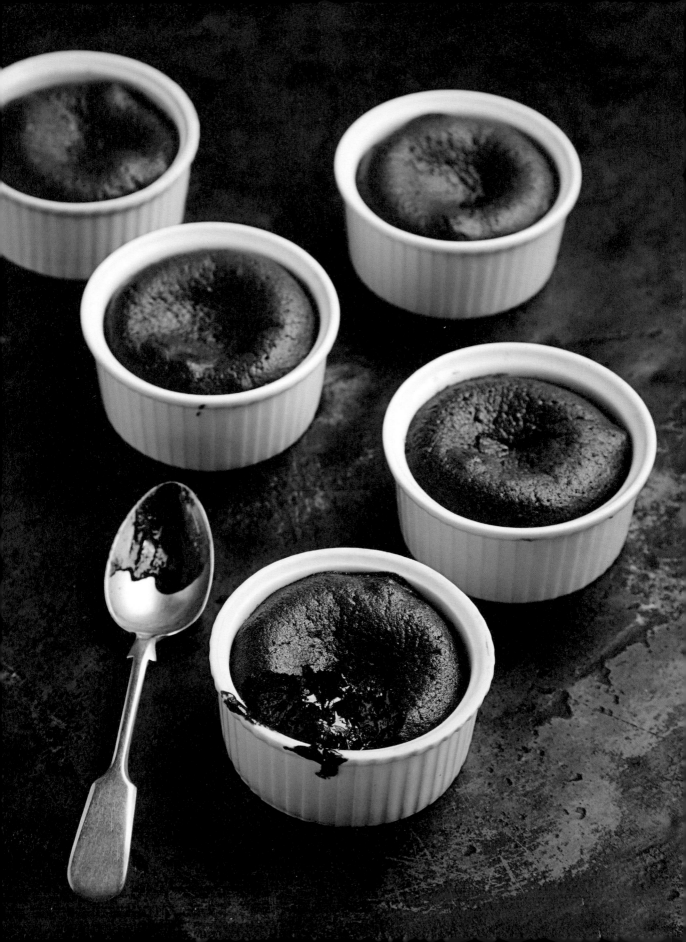

BREAKFAST

I'm not a fasting fascist. I have breakfast pretty often. How do I decide? Usually it's based on whether I have time. I know that any good diet guru will tell you to "create some me-time to nourish yourself properly". Great, if you can: go ahead and do that. But your children/wife/husband/cat will object most days. If you can manage to briefly gather your thoughts, it's worth thinking about the coming day. Are you moving house or appearing in court? Job interview? Early start? Have breakfast. You can judge. For many readers, breakfast will always be the most important meal of the day and whatever I say won't change that for you. But do factor these early calories into your daily count (see page 20).

THE CEREAL MYTH

The *New York Times* commissioned a survey of 'regular people' and nutritionists to look at the mismatch between what the public and the experts thought was healthy. Granola was the main mismatch. Even Americans don't eat cheeseburgers because they think they're healthy.

But people really believe granola is healthy. Now I've done all I can to talk about carbs and not having breakfast, but that isn't for everyone. I've also been brave and honest about my irregular attempts at breakfast. But the one thing I am certain of is that losing weight will be harder if you buy your breakfast cereal in a box – granola or not. Unless you desperately need the free toy or the table decoration that a mass-produced cereal box may offer, then don't buy the stuff. Instead make our recipe. It's much better for you.

BACON & EGGS

I know meat is said to cause cancer (but the risks of this are usually overstated) and that eggs have a lot of cholesterol (but they're actually reducing your risk of heart disease). This is my desert island breakfast. It doesn't leave me sluggish, it feels like a treat and it's far healthier than you'd think (provided you don't add toast or a bunch of other sundries).

2–3 rashers of the best bacon you can afford
Those poor pigs have a really dismal time in the industrial farms. Try to get organic, local pork, ideally from a pig with a name, some friends and access to a tennis court.

2 eggs
Again, buy the fanciest eggs you can afford. It's fun being a chicken on a good farm. Lots of grass, no foxes, few responsibilities. It's really dismal being one on a bad farm. Also, mass-produced industrial eggs aren't good for you in the same way. I can't back this claim up with a huge amount of high-quality science (see earlier grumble about nutrition research, page 13), but I'm sure it's true. Even if you only believe me about one of these points, you should still buy decent eggs.

Throw the bacon in a dry frying pan. Cook until it's crunchy in some places and sticky in others. Shove to one side.

Crack 2 eggs into the hot bacon fat. Turn them over if you like. (You don't really need directions for this part, I'm just making a point that it's easy and now – mainly – fantasizing about bacon and eggs.) Do this shirtless or in your pyjamas – not in your work clothing, depending on how sensual you want the experience to be.

Throw on a plate. Chuck the pan in the sink for later. Pour a cup of tea or coffee in a frenzied hurry. Scoff. Wipe the grease from your face. You're ready to face the day. (Put on a shirt.)

FAT (G): 5.2
PROTEIN (G): 9.8
SUGAR (G): 11.5
FIBRE (G): 7
CALORIES: 275
SERVES: 2

This is a great alternative to porridge if you don't have time to cook something in the morning. It only takes 5 minutes to throw together the night before, then simply grab and go in the morning. This is a filling, nutrient-dense breakfast.

OVERNIGHT OATS

For the oats
100g porridge oats (try steel-cut oats here to avoid the madness of cooking them)
1 tbsp seeds, or chopped nuts
40g raspberries, roughly mashed with the back of a fork
1 tsp vanilla extract
1 tsp ground cinnamon
juice of ½ lemon
175ml milk, plus more if needed (optional)
175ml water
2 tsp honey

Optional toppings
grated apple
mixed berries
orange segments
granola
nut butter
natural yogurt

In a bowl or food container, mix together all the ingredients for the oats. Leave in the fridge overnight.

When you're ready to eat, add your favourite toppings, stir and loosen up with a little milk or water if necessary. Microwave if you're not as tough as the Scottish…

FAT (G): 5.4
PROTEIN (G): 10
SUGAR (G): 5.2
FIBRE (G): 5
CALORIES: 241
SERVES: 2

Porridge is easy, inexpensive, packed full of fibre and will fuel you for the morning. The dieting programmes my twin brother Chris makes on other TV channels highly recommend it and I agree with him. It seems to be good for gut health and good for cholesterol. I say "seems", because it's not like any pharmaceutical company has commissioned a billion-pound trial of the stuff controlled against placebo, nor are the world's most enthusiastic consumers of porridge – the Scottish – a great example of slender well-being. But still.

PERFECT PORRIDGE

100g porridge oats
300ml water
200ml milk
pinch of salt

Bring the oats, water, milk and salt to a light simmer and leave to cook for 10 minutes, stirring regularly; this helps create a creamy texture. Serve topped with a handful of home-made granola or fruit, nuts and seeds of your choice and a good drizzle of honey.

VARIATIONS

Use steel-cut oats. I confess I'm too impatient for these most of the time. But they are really delicious if you can be bothered and they're the cheapest gourmet food you can get. They usually come in a nice tin that you need a screwdriver to open and that makes you feel like Mrs Beeton. What are they? Well, the quick 'rolled' oats you usually get have been crushed flat by something resembling a steam-roller, so they cook very quickly. The steel-cut alternatives have been chopped up in what I picture to be some unbelievably cool-looking steam punk-type Victorian machinery powered by a steam engine and leather belt. They're not crushed, so they cook agonisingly slowly. Soak them overnight (see page 177), or use a rice cooker.

Add 1 mashed banana and 1 tsp ground cinnamon to the porridge while cooking.

Add a handful of berries to the porridge while cooking and top with a spoonful of yogurt.

Stir through 2 tsp cocoa powder and the finely grated zest of an unwaxed orange. This is (obviously) a Georgie tip. Frankly we should all be like Georgie. It's delicious and it makes porridge taste like the gold coast of Australia rather than a rainy day in Glasgow.

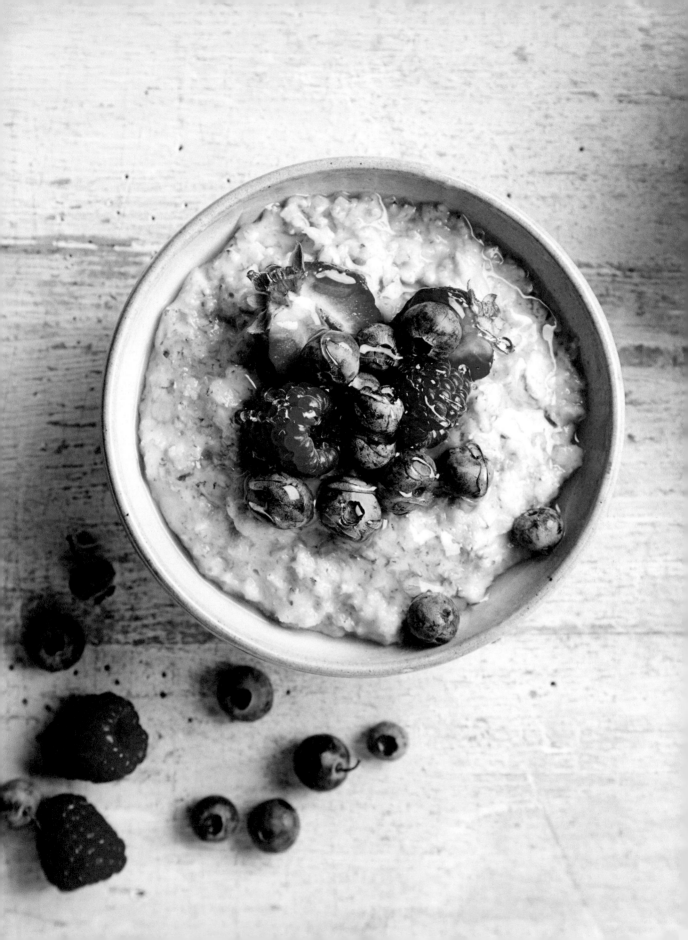

FAT (G): 24.1
PROTEIN (G): 8.1
SUGAR (G): 4.6
FIBRE (G): 4.9
CALORIES: 319
SERVES: 10–15

This stuff makes a great snack throughout the day and will keep well in an airtight container for up to 1 month. See page 175 for more on the dangers of shop-bought granola.

GRANOLA

250g oats
150g seeds
250g nuts, roughly chopped
2 tsp ground cinnamon
2 tsp vanilla extract
pinch of salt
150ml sunflower or coconut oil
50g honey
1 egg white
100g dried fruit, chopped

Preheat the oven to 160°C/gas mark 3.

In a large bowl, mix together all the ingredients except the dried fruit. Spread the mixture out on a large baking tray and bake in the oven for 35–40 minutes, mixing a couple of times during cooking so it browns evenly.

Remove from the oven and allow to cool before adding the dried fruit and mixing well. Store in an airtight container.

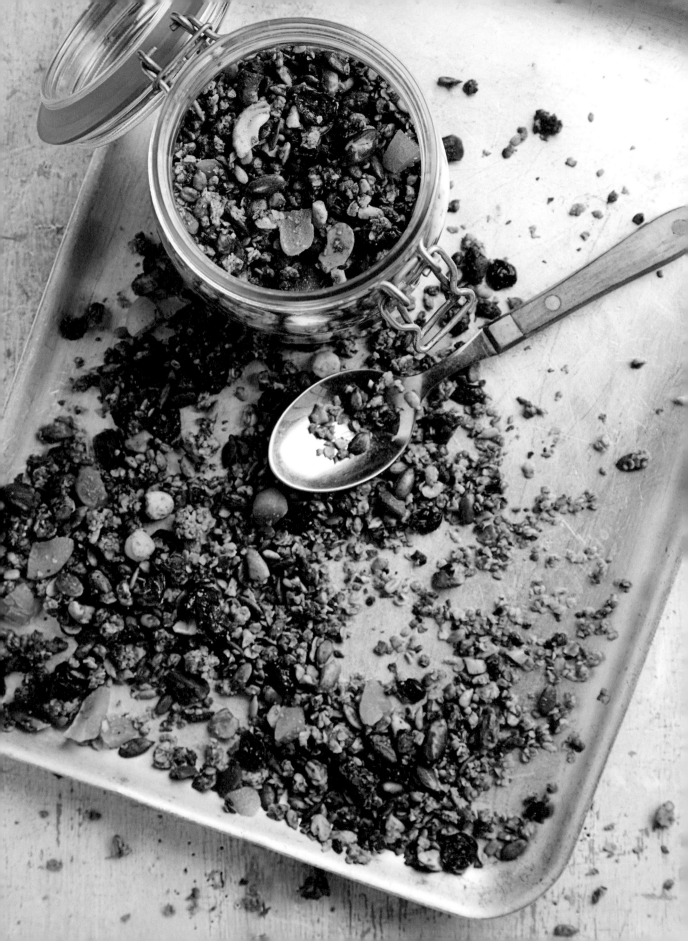

FAT (G): 13
PROTEIN (G): 16.9
SUGAR (G): 1.8
FIBRE (G): 1.6
CALORIES: 199
SERVES: 2

Eggs are good for you. I don't really believe that any one food is totally good for you, but eggs are as close as it gets. In a pinch you could live off them alone for a long time; they're a pretty complete food. They're packed with nutrients that really do seem proven to improve your heart health and brain and they fill you up.

BREAKFAST SCRAMBLE

4 eggs
50g ricotta
salt and pepper
100g spinach, roughly chopped
knob of unsalted butter
100g chestnut mushrooms, sliced

> "Cheese is good for you. Please ask anyone who disagrees to contact me directly."

In a small bowl, whisk the eggs and ricotta and season well with salt and pepper.

Place the spinach into a separate bowl and pour over just enough boiling water to cover it, then leave it for a couple of minutes to wilt. Melt the butter in a saucepan and fry the mushrooms until golden. Meanwhile, drain the spinach really well, getting as much moisture out as possible. Add the spinach and the egg mixture to the pan with the mushrooms and scramble just long enough to cook the eggs. Serve immediately.

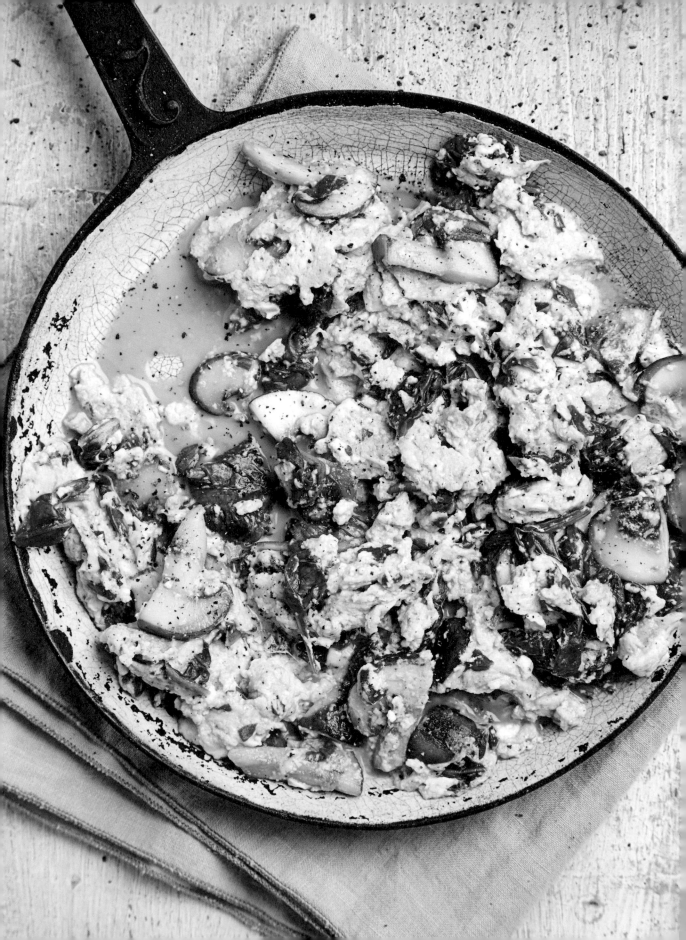

FAT (G): 8
PROTEIN (G): 10.1
SUGAR (G): 4.5
FIBRE (G): 4.6
CALORIES: 230
SERVES: 2

What am I doing recommending pancakes in a diet book? Well, make them at the weekend or go for a long walk afterwards. And don't eat too many. These are much better for you than normal pancakes, so you're still winning: they have a lower glycaemic index and far more fibre and nutrients. The pancakes keep well, too, so you can make a bigger batch to eat during the week ahead. The sweet potato helps hold the mixture together, meaning there's no need to add flour; it also adds a natural sweetness.

SWEET POTATO PANCAKES

120g cooked sweet potato (I bake a whole potato for 45 minutes, then weigh out the flesh)
2 eggs
50g oats
pinch of salt
½ tsp baking powder
knob of unsalted butter

To serve
smoked salmon, lemon and crème fraîche
OR
berries, natural yogurt and honey

In a bowl, mash the sweet potato until smooth. Add the eggs, oats, salt and baking powder and mix well. Heat the butter in a frying pan over a medium heat.

Spoon the mixture into the pan (about 1 heaped tbsp per pancake) and spread it out a little with the back of the spoon to shape into a circle. Cook for 4–5 minutes before flipping and cooking the other side. Be patient while you cook the first side of the pancake: you want to ensure it is firm enough to flip without falling apart.

For a savoury breakfast, serve with smoked salmon, lemon and crème fraîche, or for a sweet option serve with berries, yogurt and honey. Do NOT drown them in maple or – worse – golden syrup.

This mixture and cooked pancakes will keep in the fridge for 3–4 days.

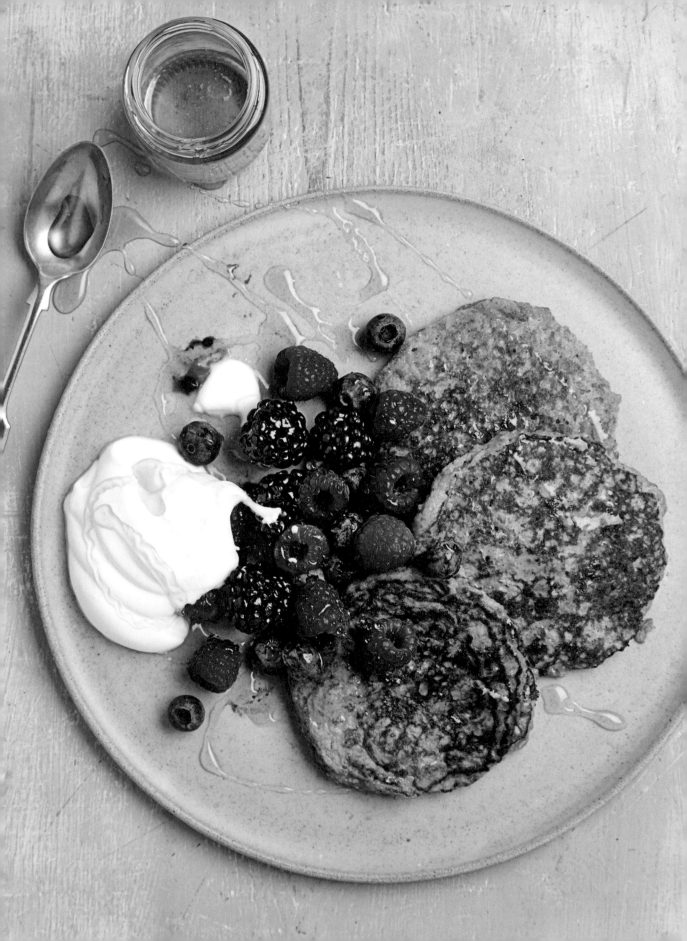

FAT (G): 10.8
PROTEIN (G): 12.2
SUGAR (G): 1.1
FIBRE (G): 1
CALORIES: 154
SERVES: 2

The punchy flavours here really set you up for the day and get your digestion going. (Georgie and I have collaborated on all of these recipes and this is Georgie's delicate euphemism for "helps you poo". I thought you'd enjoy it.) It's filling without being too heavy or leaving you with those sugar lows mid-morning. It's a great speedy lunch or dinner, too.

SPINACH MASALA OMELETTE

4 eggs
salt and pepper
1 tsp garam masala
½ red chilli, chopped (I, Xand, add much more, especially if I'm up early. Some weeks it's the only time I feel alive)
2 spring onions, sliced
small knob of unsalted butter
50g spinach, chopped
lime wedges, to serve

Break the eggs into a bowl, season with salt and pepper, add the garam masala, chilli and spring onions and whisk with a fork until combined.

Melt the butter in a medium non-stick frying pan and pour in the egg mixture. Tilt the pan and swirl the egg around the pan until it is fully coated. After 30 seconds, when the omelette has started to set, push the edges into the middle – this helps the omelette cook more quickly and evenly – do this a couple of times and then sprinkle over the spinach. Leave the omelette to cook for another minute or so until the top is just set.

Fold the omelette in half and carefully wiggle it on to a plate. Serve with the lime juice squeezed over the top.

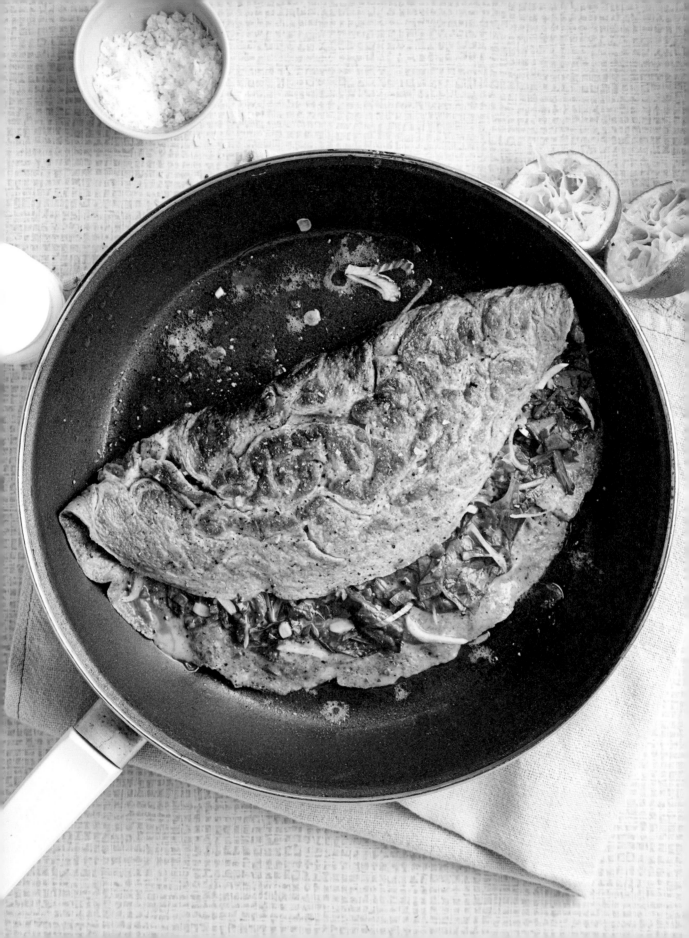

FAT (G): 25.7
PROTEIN (G): 27.3
SUGAR (G): 0.9
FIBRE (G): 1.1
CALORIES: 354
SERVES: 2

This is a simple, one-tray breakfast, perfect for the weekend, especially if you have guests. It's ideal for a weekday only if you're not as chronically late as me. The addition of spinach packs in some good vegetable nutrients and much-needed fibre, but also creates a clever nest to bake the eggs in without having to add any oil. (For more baked eggs recipes, see page 145).

GEORGINA'S FANCY BAKED GREEN EGGS & BACON

4 rashers of streaky bacon
100g spinach
4 eggs
salt and pepper

Preheat the oven to 200°C/gas mark 6.

Lay the bacon at one side of a large baking tray and roast in the oven for 6–7 minutes until just starting to crisp up.

Remove the tray from the oven and place the spinach on the other side of the tray, making a slight indentation in the centre. Crack the eggs into the indentation, season well with salt and pepper and place back in the oven for a further 5 minutes, or until the egg whites are just set and the bacon is crispy. Serve immediately.

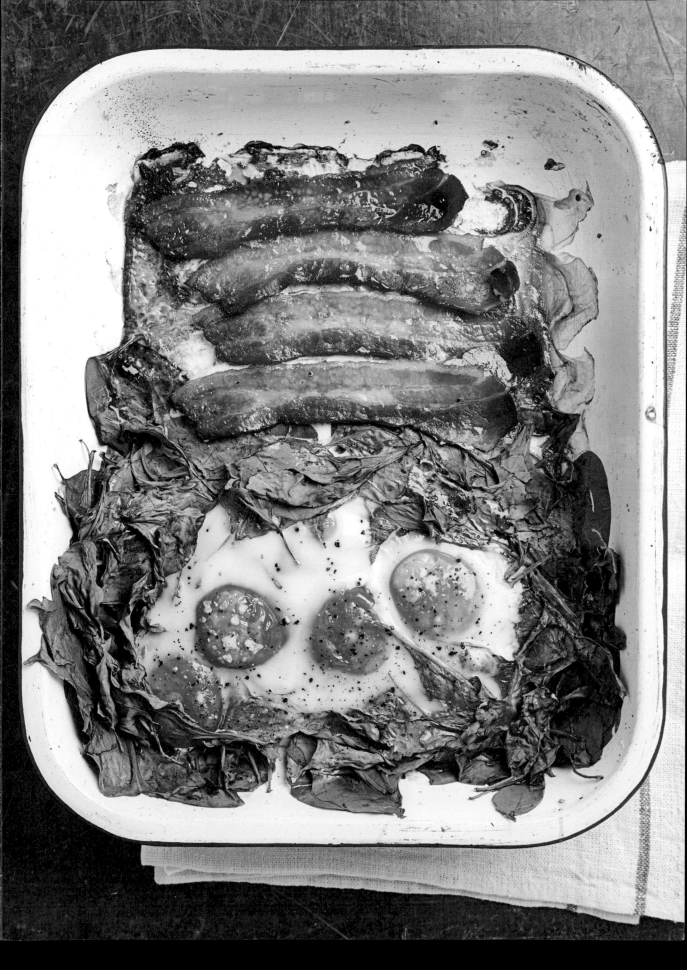

INDEX

Publishing director: Sarah Lavelle
Creative director: Helen Lewis
Editor: Céline Hughes
Art direction & design concept: Smith & Gilmour
Photography: Louise Hagger and Colin Bell
Food stylist: Georgina Davies
Props stylist: Jenny Iggledon
Production: Stephen Lang, Vincent Smith

First published in 2016 by Quadrille Publishing
Pentagon House, 52–54 Southwark Street,
London SE1 1UN

Quadrille Publishing is an
imprint of Hardie Grant
www.hardiegrant.com.au
www.quadrille.co.uk

Reprinted in 2016 (twice), 2017
10 9 8 7 6 5 4

Cataloguing in Publication Data: a catalogue record
for this book is available from the British Library.

978 1 84949 951 4

Printed in Italy

ACKNOWLEDGEMENTS

Molly Wilkof who wrote and read and re-read and stayed up very late.

Brother Chris for reassurance and science and clear thinking even when you were extremely busy.

My mother and father and Brother JJ for being wonderful at so many mealtimes.

My amazing co-presenter Hala El-Shafie, the best – and my favourite – dietitian.

Kurt Seywald, Ben Gale and Natasha Bondy from Little Gem for being relentlessly cheerful and meticulous and working so hard on the show.

Martin Brake for the hair transplant (and crystal clear sound).

Matilda Hay and Chris Clarke for fantastic research and good humour.

Sharon Newson – you're an inspiration to anyone wanting to change their life.

The Whites: Dylan, Nicky, Tash and Suzannah for your lessons in how to be a family.

Miranda and Kate at ROAR for being the absolute best people in the world.

Céline and the team at Quadrille for all your fantastic work and guidance and help pushing me along.

Alexander Greene, my dear friend, who helped fatten me up and slim me down.

Georgina, for going miles above and beyond and being so creative over long distances.

All the contributors of *How to Lose Weight Well* for being so honest and game to try anything.

The mistakes are my own, the good bits are everyone else's and the funny bits are Molly Wilkof's.

ABOUT GEORGINA DAVIES

Georgina Davies is a London-based chef, food stylist and recipe writer who is passionate about delicious, healthy food made from fresh and seasonal ingredients. Her extensive knowledge of nutrition – gleaned from numerous cookery courses and a nutrition course – forms the basis of her recipes, which are balanced without compromising on flavour.